stuttering: successes and failures in therapy

Actual Case Histories as Reported by Authorities

These reports sponsored and published by

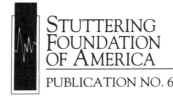

STUTTERING
FOUNDATION
OF AMERICA

PUBLICATION NO. 6

stuttering: successes and
failures in therapy
Publication No. 6

First Printing–1968
Second Printing–1970
Third Printing–1972
Fourth Printing–1975
Fifth Printing–1978
Sixth Printing–1982
Seventh Printing–1995
Eighth Printing–1997

Published by

Stuttering Foundation of America
P. O. Box 11749
Memphis, Tennessee 38111-0749

ISBN-0-933388-04-7

To The Reader:

Historically, the Stuttering Foundation of America sponsored conferences for the purpose of promoting agreement among eminent speech pathologists on matters related to stuttering. One of the earlier conferences was on the subject of a most important aspect of treatment—the nature of the interaction between the clinician and his or her client.

This book, which was out of print for a year, was the product of that conference. Although its origin was some years ago, the information is as revealing and enlightening in 1995 as it was originally in 1968; and we have reprinted a new edition because of numerous requests for it.

Those whose names are listed on the following pages were first invited to direct themselves to the question "What are the personal behavioral characteristics that lead to success or failure in stuttering?" All of them were asked to outline two case studies: one which they viewed as success; the other failure.

In each case they were to include enough description of the client, the circumstances of therapy, and the therapeutic process to allow the others to see what kind of people were in therapy, how they as therapists saw their own roles and where they thought they had failed or succeeded. In this book we are publishing these true case histories, although fictitious names have been used, and we believe you will find them most interesting. It may be reassuring for some to know that experts often fail to attain reasonable success.

After the case histories were written, these same authorities met in a week's conference to discuss these cases and uncover some generalizations about the effects of the clinical relationship upon the success or failure of therapy. The notes taken from the conference discussions are included in this book.

JANE FRASER

For the Stuttering Foundation of America
Memphis, Tennessee

Participants

Joseph G. Sheehan, Ph.D.

Professor of psychology, University of California, Los Angeles. Diplomate in clinical psychology, American Board Examiners in Professional Psychology. Editor, "Stuttering Research and Therapy."

Alastair A. Stunden, Ph.D.

Clinical psychologist and speech pathologist; assistant professor speech pathology and co-director, Speech Clinic, California State College at Los Angeles; consultant in special education and clinical psychology, Los Angeles County Schools.

Charles Van Riper, Ph.D.

Distinguished Professor Emeritus and formerly Head, Department of Speech Pathology and Audiology, Western Michigan University. Honors of the American Speech-Language-Hearing Association and formerly Councilor and Associate Editor. Author, "The Treatment of Stuttering."

Dean Williams, Ph.D.

Professor Speech Pathology and Audiology, University of Iowa. Fellow and formerly Councilor, American Speech-Language-Hearing Association. Editorial Board, Journal of Communication Disorders.

Malcolm Fraser

Executive Director, Speech Foundation of America.

Participants

Stanley Ainsworth, Ph.D., Chairman

Alumni Foundation distinguished professor emeritus of speech correction, University of Georgia. Past President and Executive Vice-President, American Speech-Language-Hearing Association.

Lon Emerick, Ph.D.

Professor, Department Speech Pathology and Audiology, Speech and Hearing Clinic, Northern Michigan University.

Hugo H. Gregory, Ph.D.

Professor and Head, Speech and Language Pathology, Northwestern University. Fellow, American Speech-Language-Hearing Association. Editor, "Learning Theory and Stuttering Therapy."

Harold L. Luper, Ph.D., Editor

Professor and Head, Department of Audiology and Speech Pathology, University of Tennessee. Fellow and formerly Vice-President for Administration, American Speech-Language-Hearing Association.

Frank Robinson, Ph.D.

Professor and formerly chairman, Department of Speech Pathology and Audiology, Western Michigan University. Author, "Introduction to Stuttering." Fellow, American Speech-Language-Hearing Association.

TABLE OF CONTENTS
Part I

STANLEY AINSWORTH

    A Clinical Success: Lynne................................ 11

    A Clinical Failure: Bill.................................. 16

LON EMERICK

    A Clinical Success: Mark................................ 21

    A Clinical Failure: Sherrie.............................. 32

HUGO GREGORY

    A Clinical Success: Cora................................ 41

    A Clinical Failure: Fred................................. 47

HAROLD L. LUPER

    A Clinical Success: Steve............................... 55

    A Clinical Failure: Elaine............................... 59

FRANK B. ROBINSON

    A Clinical Success: Louise.............................. 65

    A Clinical Failure: Harry............................... 72

JOSEPH SHEEHAN

    A Clinical Success: Leonard............................ 77

    A Clinical Failure: Rudolf.............................. 82

ALASTAIR A. STUNDEN

    A Clinical Success: Alex................................ 87

    A Clinical Failure: Arthur.............................. 91

C. VAN RIPER

    A Clinical Success: Don................................ 99

    A Clinical Failure: Melinda.............................121

DEAN E. WILLIAMS

    A Clinical Success: John................................125

    A Clinical Failure: Susan...............................131

Part II

NOTES FROM THE CONFERENCE DISCUSSIONS........135

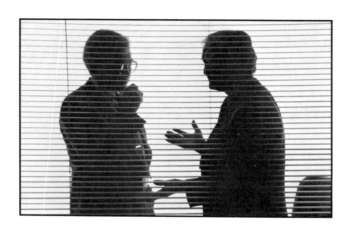

Introduction

Before you begin to read the case studies and generalizations, those of us who participated in the conference would like to point out some of the restrictions which we feel are inherent in the material. As we prepared our case studies, it soon became apparent that what we were reporting were not "the facts" but our perceptions thereof. Since success and failure in stuttering therapy depend so much upon the clinician and his ability to engender growth in his clients, the task was largely one of self-scrutiny. This is always difficult. Self-confrontation is perhaps the most formidable and intricate of human undertakings. Even with detailed clinical records, our memories were admittedly subject to error and, perhaps, to retroactive embellishment. The writing and later discussions of these case studies was frequently an agonizing process. We suffered as we wrote and, again, when our mistakes were discussed by our respected colleagues. But we tried to be honest, and, in so doing, we felt we learned a great deal about ourselves, our vulnerabilities, our strengths, and what is more important, about the therapeutic process.

We were also concerned that, in reviewing one's successes and failures, in casting the cold eye upon our craft and in dissecting the bones so thoroughly, the process would leave us only with barren matter. We feared that such a process would dry up the springs of clinical creativity. It did not. It was a lively and productive series of sessions.

We hope the reader will not view these accounts of therapy as representing what we typically do with all the stutterers we treat. We selected these particular case studies because we felt they would stimulate intense discussion. We did not choose them to display our professional competence or merely to expound a theoretical point of view. What we have assembled here are those successes and failures which we felt would reveal the hidden processes underlying clinical judgement, those that determined what the therapist did and why he did it.

It is important to note that during our analysis and discussion of these cases, there was the implied assumption that therapy is an interaction process, that it involves an exchange and relationship between two people. At times, we fixated on the specific details of treatment, but wherever possible, we soon returned to the focus of the conference—what were we like? how did our role affect the client? how did our client's self perceptions affect us?

PART I

Case Studies of Successes and Failures

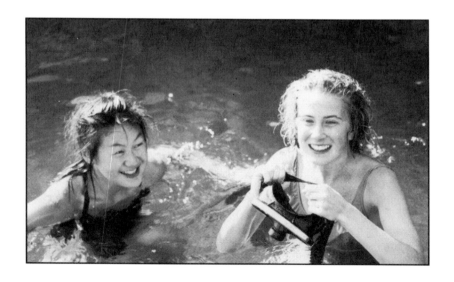

A CLINICAL SUCCESS: LYNNE
CLINICIAN: STANLEY AINSWORTH

introduction

The following summary seems to be deceptively simple. The haunting thought arises that most of the successful cases have been equally "simple" and the unsuccessful ones have been "complex." Girls, in particular, have seemed to fall into those who progress quickly and easily—or are hopelessly resistant to change.

background

Lynne was 21 years old when I first saw her. She had been referred by her major professor because he noted some difficulty during her student teaching in high school English during the fall quarter of her senior year in college.

The initial examination and subsequent sessions revealed frequent hesitations and blocking, but only mild secondary reactions most of the time. The eye blinks and head movements were noticeable only on the worst blocks. Substitutions on feared words were reported. She talked softly most of the time, but there was no noticeable reluctance to communicate. She reported much more frequent and severe stuttering intermittently in situations other than the clinic.

The history of her problem was fairly representative of a great many stutterers. She had "always" stuttered. She received some "help" in the first and second grades. Instructions included telling her to read a lot and to sing words instead of speaking them. The stuttering became much more severe in the third, fourth, and fifth grades. She remembers herself as a "pitiful case" and that at times she "couldn't say anything." However, the speech had been getting better until she began her student teaching. During her freshman year at another university, she took the fundamentals of speech course with no particular difficulty except for some help with "pronunciation." There was a family history of stuttering. The mother stuttered about as severely as Lynne, and two uncles had a similar difficulty. There was no history of specific trauma to relate to her speech problems, although the possible separation of her brother and his wife was possibly one factor in the increase of stuttering at the time of the examination.

She was unusually aware of her stuttering and could anticipate blocks with considerable consistency. She felt that she could reliably precipitate stuttering if she thought about a word, particularly if it began with one of her feared sounds. Frequently, she did not talk in classes or groups for fear of stuttering or—as therapy later brought out—because she felt that what she had to offer was not worthwhile. In social situations, she was not "bothered" by stuttering, although her sorority sisters and friends sometimes told her to "stop stuttering"—which actually produced more fluency at times. Some days she was free of any noticeable blocking. Telephoning was difficult for her, particularly when she initiated the call and had to say her name. She had attempted to improve her speech in various ways—such as taking a deep breath, lowering her voice, clenching her hands, forcing the word out, moving her head, and substituting words—but had given up most of them as unsuccessful.

Lynne was an attractive girl who had many signs that she was adjusting reasonably well socially. In the sorority she was well accepted, but she avoided leadership roles. Scholastically she was well above average. She was engaged at the time of the initial interview and was married in the June following her senior year—an "ideal" arrangement sought by many girls! There certainly were no apparent signs of "emotional maladjustments."

discussion of therapy

The formal sessions with Lynne totaled 21 of one to one and one-half hours each during the winter and spring quarters of her senior year in college. Subsequently, it was possible to provide intermittent support and informal therapy because she continued in graduate school. She was dismissed as "satisfactory" at the end of the spring quarter.

Initial conferences were used to determine further details concerning the characteristics of her stuttering and situations which seemed to be related to the increase in stuttering at the present time.

Three sources of tension or pressure in recent months were determined. These were: the student teaching; an impending separation of her older brother and his wife, both of whom were very close to her; and her impending marriage. At the close of the initial session, an underlying factor seemed to be revealed. She noted that she was quiet and reserved many times because of deep feelings of unworthiness and of the value of any contribution which she might make. On the basis of this evaluation, it was made clear that therapy would aim to alter the frame of reference which she might have regarding disturbing incidents, to determine the ways in which her feelings were related to the increase in stuttering in specific situations, and to change specific behaviors which would in turn affect the feelings. We made a detailed analysis of the fears created by the many situations. In the third and fourth sessions we began to help her become aware of her definite personality assets, in contrast to the fears and insecurities and unworthiness which she felt.

It became apparent that she had a great deal of shame and guilt concerning her home and self. The house was one which had been built during war time and was modern in appearance, but the entire neighborhood was becoming rather run down. All houses in the neighborhood were small. She had spent considerable time in the home of her older brother and his wife. She felt that she needed to conceal what she viewed as an inferior social status from her sorority sisters. Therefore, she had never invited anyone to go home with her. The possibility of her brother and his wife separating was something which bothered her, but she had already been away long enough so that this was something that she was willing to accept. There was not any particular history of great deal of conflict in the home while she and her two younger brothers were growing up. She expressed some guilt feelings concerning her attitudes toward her family.

One of the areas upon which we were able to focus involved the relationships with the prospective in-laws. Nearly every week there were instances which provided a basis for self understanding, since they lived a short distance from the University, and she frequently spent weekends with them. Most of the outward relationships were excellent. The family was devoted to church going, and although Lynne had not been brought up with strict church attendance, she was willing to follow the pattern of the in-laws. Her own reactions to very simple and everyday occurrences was revealing. She felt that she could never do anything to help around the house that would be acceptable. It became clear that this was not due to any implied or actual criticism but rather her own feelings of inadequacy even to such simple things as washing dishes. During these periods when she was alone with her prospective mother-in-law and attempting to help, she found her speech getting much worse. At other times, she was unable to express any kind of opposition or difference from what the family said or suggested, even though she strongly disagreed.

As she began to realize exactly how she felt about herself in contrast to her awareness of her assets and potentialities, definite steps were taken to alter behavior directly. At first this was only on a very tentative and moderate basis, but gradually began to affect more and more of her behavior. She managed to strike a nice balance between standing up for herself and not becoming defensive or unpleasantly aggressive. In other words, she was able to maintain her generally good relationships with people, but still assert her self respect. She began to stand up for herself and to express her opinions. She paid an exorbitant amount for some clothes, but then was helped to realize that this was done to impress her friends. Very soon this kind of insight was reached many times without any direct assignments except those which she selected for herself from general discussion. She worked continuously on her problem between sessions. This was reflected in the detail with which she could report on what had taken place. At the same time she continued to participate in the multiplicity of activities of attending school, preparing for a wedding, and being involved in the sorority activities of the final quarter of the senior year. Fortunately for the pattern of therapy, there was a very close relationship between the amount of stuttering and the depth of feelings of inadequacy or inferiority. These feelings were subtle enough so that sometimes she was not aware that she was operating in her old pattern. She learned to use the stuttering as a clue to the existence of these feelings. Stuttering reduced rapidly in nearly all situations. Occasionally, when stuttering seemed to "come back" she became adept at analyzing the basis for this. This immediately brought some drop in stuttering, but it occasionally reduced only gradually over a period of two or three days. This process, however, immediately relieved her anxiety about the existence of the stuttering.

The progress report for the second quarter of therapy reports the following results. "She apparently is adjusting very well and stuttering has been materially reduced. It was revived temporarily in one instance during which she responded to praise with more stuttering. She became aware of what was happening and was able to readjust and thus reduce the stuttering. It would appear that she is, for all practical purposes, a normal speaker."

follow-up

After marrying in June, she continued in graduate school for one calendar year and finished a Master's degree in child development. This provided an opportunity for intermittent checks with her concerning the status of her feelings and speech. Reasonably good fluency continued to hold up very well except for occasional lapses which she was able to analyze. The speech continued to contain some very mild blockages which most people ignored. At the end of a year of training, she moved to a nearby city and has made telephone calls and written letters since that time. Periods of unusual stress sometimes bring some return of symptoms but to a lesser degree than formerly, and they are reasonably temporary in nature.

discussion

Lynne had essential readiness to do something about her situation. She had had enough social and personal success and an awareness of this to form a basis to tackle some of her feelings of unworthiness and inadequacy. Furthermore, she was willing to talk about herself and her feelings without becoming too deeply involved emotionally in the process itself. My own role as a therapist is somewhat difficult to describle. In one sense, the most important contributions were of a passive and permissive character rather than anything concrete and positive. On the other hand, suggestions for analyses, interpretations, and direct assignments were provided at appropriate times. Success, I believe, was due to a fortunate combination of several procedures that allowed key elements to emerge without an imposition by the therapist of a preconceived idea as to what should be done. In other words, the case was ready to do something, and I kept out of her way so that she could do it. I did not impose a standard regime, such as assignments and controls of blocking, because this did not appear to be necessary. In this sense, the important role here was that of a catalyst to help her become aware of the discrepancy between some of her feelings and the essential reality. At the same time I provided opportunities for her to discuss her attempts to remedy her behavior and her feelings in an atmosphere which was supportive and mildly directive.

At the same time, this review of the case has made certain inadequacies very apparent. These inadequacies did not have any derogatory effects on therapy, fortunately. One is the very few notes that were taken about the therapy sessions. Perhaps it would have been well to have had tape recordings, because the key elements threaded through a welter of mundane events and discussions. It might have been possible to have gone back and picked these out if a complete record had been kept. On the other hand, this freedom from attempts to utilize her for learning purposes may have had a fundamental effect on the relationships established between the therapist and Lynne. This raises an important question. To what degree do the efforts to utilize a case in concrete and specific ways for training of the therapist himself or other therapists affect the fundamental therapeutic process?

Another outcome of this case was revealing over a period of time. The ease with which she progressed resulted in an attempt to utilize very similar methods with subsequent stutterers, particularly girls who probably had some of her basic characteristics. The efforts were a definite failure, except in one very brief case that seemed to arrive at some insights that were not at all clear to me but seemed to take care of the situation. In other cases, the direct relationships between self concepts and stuttering were not as apparent. And, again, I became impressed with the need for individual adaptation of therapy.

A CLINICAL FAILURE: BILL
CLINICIAN: STANLEY AINSWORTH

introduction

This attempt to present an adequate summary of my therapy with Bill is as frustrating as my year of working with him. There is the same "quicksilver" quality in attempting to discuss what happened as I experienced then—more than thirteen years ago. The fact that some of my conclusions were proved reasonably correct in the subsequent years is of little satisfaction in face of the failure to rescue a lonely individual from his own personal desert island.

description and background

Bill was referred to the clinic by his dormitory counselor during his first quarter as a freshman at the University. He demonstrated severe stuttering with many secondary reactions used simultaneously or in sequence in a variety of combinations. This complex process plus some distorted sounds in non-stuttered speech made him difficult to understand at times. Talking with him was always a slow process with many distracting elements. There were tic-like head movements even during silence and a history of rheumatic fever at age eleven. He had "always stuttered" and did not know if the stuttering was worse after the rheumatic fever. He felt that his speech had improved since he was in grade school. (The accuracy of this judgment is difficult to assess). He admitted to some social timidity—an understatement, because he had practically no social life. Little family background was detailed in initial visits. (It was hard to get much important or meaningful information from him). He was the only stutterer in a family of seven children and in the small high school which he attended. His ambitions were to get an advanced degree and to become a sales engineer or a certified public accountant.

discussion of therapy

During his freshman year, from November through June, I recorded 35 one hour (or longer) sessions with Bill. (He subsequently received 207 additional speech therapy sessions—mostly individual—during the years that it took him to complete his Bachelor's degree).

In the first quarter, I first tried to help him understand stuttering as a form of learned behavior—a comparatively frequent disfluency that had become intensified and complicated by the efforts to prevent, avoid, or conceal the interruption and by various feelings associated with the process. We tried to determine his degree of awareness concerning his secondary reactions and his feelings and to follow this with conscious imitation of the secondary patterns. We also tried to modify his stuttering by using the bounce pattern. In general, results in regard to all these were limited and unsatisfactory. Sound substitutions and distortions and lack of awareness of sounds or how they were made interfered with conscious efforts to modify his speech. He felt the bounce pattern helped him relax—but he was nearly always optimistic in a generalized sort of way. There was practically no insight about his feelings or the basis for them—except that a lot of things made him "nervous." In addition, I tried to pin down any neurological basis for any of his speech difficulties. The visiting psychiatrist, after relatively limited testing, reported normal neurological responses—that the "tic" was functional and related to the stuttering. An EEG could not be arranged.

In the first month of the second quarter, Bill's counselor called me to report that he had failed French and mathematics in the fall quarter and was repeating them. In February, Bill went to the University physician because of an inability to sleep. The physician referred Bill to the Psychology Clinic—which, in turn, asked me for a report that included the following kinds of statements.

"In regard to stuttering therapy, Bill shows considerable passiveness. He is very ready to nod his head and indicate that he understands. Subsequent questions reveal that his understanding is extremely superficial. He is always willing to do what he is told, but frequently confuses assignments. He always does something, however. He is inclined to do no more than what he had been assigned and has shown no initiative in helping himself to correct his problem of stuttering.

"There is some question of his ability to handle college work, particularly at the level to which he aspires . . .

"On the verbal level he does not indicate much insight into his problem. His general attitude is that he is getting along fine. He does not resist any attempt to help him or to probe into his problems, but merely presents a front of 'There is nothing the matter . . .' An example of his tendency to cover and ignore inadequacy is illustrated by his French course. As part of the session on phonetic awareness of speech sounds, I asked if he had any trouble with French. His answer was, 'No,'—that he was getting along fine."

I recommended counseling. Bill was assigned to a psychologist who saw him several times. The level of counseling was questionable. The psychologist was satisfied that the answer to Bill's problem was simple because he had talked fluently in some sessions after being told to relax, slow down his walking, and take hot showers at night (as reported to me by the psychologist).

In therapy, we concentrated on reduction of tensions and fears in various situations and on techniques for handling blocks more effectively. Results were very limited even in the clinic situation. He did not seem to grasp the concept of controlling stuttering.

The spring quarter was a repetition. Some control was established at times in the clinic, but it was not maintained consistently and broke down when any kind of pressure was applied. Review of basic goals was frequently necessary, negative practice was not done consistently, he still attacked words in phonetically impossible ways, assignments were not done correctly. Periodic attempts at a counseling approach got nowhere.

follow up

Bill continued in therapy for most of his years in and out of college. Failures and low grades made him repeat many courses. He often came to the clinic for informal conferences even when not enrolled in therapy. A review of progress reports indicates that more sophisticated controls were attempted (preparatory sets, cancellations, etc.), and an effort was made to move toward a more objective attitude, to become more active socially, to have him assume more responsibility for his own therapy. The last report (more than six years after the first) stated that there was some improvement in frequency of use of speech controls during therapy sessions, but no over-all consistency in decrease of stuttering severity nor any general increase in habitual use of techniques for decreasing severity of blocks. In the meantime, he had received testing and guidance for more realistic vocational objectives. One quarter devoted entirely to a counseling approach in the clinic demonstrated no progress. He was finally turned over to psychology and psychiatry.

Following graduation, Bill obtained work as a stock clerk which allowed him to work in a secluded and protected environment. He began therapy with a psychiatrist but anticipated that it would not take long to solve his problems.

Five years after graduation, a letter from him reported that his job did not have much of a future but he was thinking of becoming a composer. (He had shown an interest in this while still in college). He felt that he was learning more about himself. He gave credit to one student clinician for helping him to acquire more self confidence and to realize that his "real trouble" was deeper than his speech. (However, this student had worked with him four years before he graduated). He was still having depressions, but they didn't "hurt him very much," and he knew that the future would be much better.

discussion

Where to begin? It is hard to separate my year of work with him from what I have learned about him since then. An enumeration of what I see as my own inadequacies in working with Bill would not present an accurate picture of what was important. For one thing, my therapeutic limitations were definitely related to my perceptions of Bill and his needs. My basic attitudes toward him were not conducive to much constructive activity on my part. I was too sorry for him. I soon considered him to be hopeless. I felt that he had a thin veneer of pseudosophistication covering a vast shallowness—under which were submerged all the haunting inadequacies of someone with serious limitations. How could I expect him to have any capacity for important insights into his problems? (It is of little help to me to know that others were frustrated over several subsequent years and that many of my specific conclusions were apparently justified. The important thing is that my attitude precluded any solution of his problems). The severity of his symptoms did not dismay me—but their persistence in face of attempts to modify them did contribute to my convictions.

Looking back, I can see some basic ambivalences in my attitudes toward him and my understandings of his needs. First there was my awareness of his need for something deep and basic within himself. This might have been reached by a powerful combination of understanding, permissiveness, and support, but it demanded a depth of effort that I did not have the capacity for or did not wish to expend on a hopeless project. Foiled in my attempts to grasp a key factor or to achieve any important communication with him, I was pushed to the opposite—from support and understanding to an impulse to shock him into facing reality and himself. But it seemed likely that this too would fail—and only beat him down. So I withheld my psychological clubs—and not knowing what to substitute for them, I withdrew in that subtle way clinicians have—openly willing to listen and help, but by non-verbal cues, discouraging his talking to me. On the more technical side, this move on my part was expressed by an abandonment of psychological approaches and a retreat to oversimplified control of speech—essentially a mechanical approach. (At the time I thought this was a realistic appraisal of what would be successful. Perhaps it was—but it failed to help him).

Another vague but persistent awareness pushed me to use an essential withdrawal to an over-simplified approach. I was afraid he would attach himself to me and become a full-time obligation. I sensed the desperate loneliness deep within the boy. I could not try to fill this emptiness—this, at least, was a realistic judgment. Nor could I tackle the comprehensive restructuring necessary to reduce this aloneness—a decision due in part to my evaluation of his inability to do or to understand so many things.

And so, Bill was passed along to others who, I hoped, would not be as limited as I. But it looks as if he is still being "passed along."

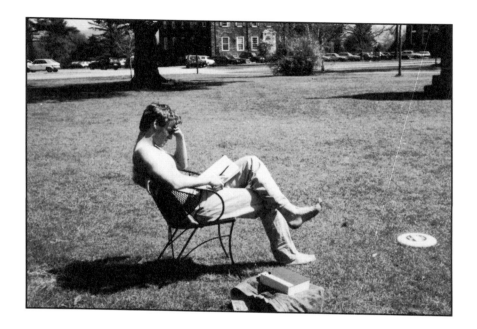

A CLINICAL SUCCESS: MARK
CLINICIAN: LON EMERICK

Not long after assuming my duties as director of a new training program in speech pathology at a small college in the upper Midwest, I received the following plea for help from a second grade teacher in the local school system:

> I realize from the article in the newspaper that you are just beginning a training program in speech, but I need help right now with one of my children. Mark stutters very badly, and his mother has asked me several times to work with him after school. I have tried, but I'm sure that I'm doing all the wrong things; anyway, it just doesn't seem to help. Would you please see him and talk with his mother?

We did see Mark and his mother later that week. Mark was a rather large, blond boy, somewhat shy and awkward but with a compelling crooked smile. He was indeed stuttering as his mother announced when she pushed him firmly before her into my office. His blocks were mainly tonic or fixative, but he came jerking and bouncing out of them with a series of inspiratory gasps accompanied by a peculiar shudder—almost like a series of rapid Moro reflexes—of his chest, neck and shoulders. During the worst of them, he covered his mouth with his hand and lowered his head. He did not have the well developed avoidances, sound fears, word fears or the elaborate covert aspects that characterize confirmed adult stutterers. But he sure was frustrated by his speech barriers. Although he still had some periods of comparative fluency, especially during vacations from school, these were becoming more and more infrequent. Mark was, in other words, at stage three in the four phase development of stuttering as described by Van Riper (1963).

According to his mother, Mark began to stutter when he was about three years old. She traced the cause for the problem back to the child's first year of life. When he was six months old, Mark had an extremely high fever of unknown etiology which precipitated a series of severe convulsions. The parents were told that the child probably had sustained "minimal brain damage" and that they should watch his development closely for signs of abnormality. Apparently, they did watch closely; they heard the disfluency known to characterize the speech of children. Mark was taken to a pediatrician, and the parents were told that Mark would grow out of "it" (Emerick and Teigland, 1965); they decided they should help him grow out of it faster by suggesting that he stop and start over again, think what he was going to say, take a deep breath—all the old home remedies for stuttering. Mark's problem had grown steadily more severe, especially since he started kindergarten. Although he was a bright boy—an I.Q. of 121 was obtained on a comprehensive intelligence measure—he was doing poorly at school; he refused to participate in oral activities and was teased by several of his classmates.

Mrs. Swenson, Mark's mother, was a physically large and psychologically dominating woman in her early forties. A teacher by profession—she held a permanent certificate in secondary education with a major in English and a minor in speech—she tended to be direct and didactic in her relationships with others. Prior to her marriage, she had taught in the local junior high school and still substituted on occasion. Each spring she promoted, directed, and judged an oral interpretation contest in the community. Mrs. Swenson enjoyed a reputation in the community as an excellent public speaker; she had served as president of the P. T. A. for four consecutive years. I did find her to be an accomplished speaker although quite rapid in rate and very complex in style; when she could use a word like "germane," "anachronistic," or "recalcitrant" she actually seemed to derive oral pleasure. As a listener, I found myself so enthralled by the pear-shaped tones, the clever epigrams, and the hand supine that, instead of responding to her message, I wanted to applaud. Mark's stuttering was, for her, both a personal and a professional failure, and she was convinced that the neighbors and teachers in the small town blamed her for the child's problem.

Mark's father was the very busy manager of a drive-in restaurant, one of a national chain that features an inexpensive hamburger. After several abortive phone calls, broken appointments and one fleeting conversation beside a sputtering grill, he finally consented to an interview in the Clinic. He came primed—the first thing he said when he arrived (ten minutes late) was: "I have a very loving relationship with my son." Yet, after discussing his relationship with Mark, it soon became apparent that Mr. Swenson preferred his eldest son who was a skilled Little League athlete at twelve. Although he told of pitching practice and other athletic activities carried out with the older son, he could think of not one thing he had done with Mark. He waved airily, dismissing this by indicating that Mark liked fishing and nature study and "Who has time for driving to the lake or chasing bugs?" Mr. Swenson refused to sit down during the interview and paced back and forth, smoking incessantly. To all my attempts to explain Mark's problem he countered, "You're the expert" and rejected any notion that he might have a role in the child's speech therapy. When asked how he reacted when Mark stuttered he said that he pretended it didn't exist and hoped that if he persisted in this behavior it might go away. As he was leaving, he remembered something and came back to pour out the following story regarding the onset of Mark's stuttering. I cannot resist reporting it:

> Every summer we go to my folks' place. They live on a small farm north of here and raise a little bit of everything. Well, this one year when Mark was three, we were there visiting while my Dad had a bunch of suckling pigs. I was going to take them over to sell to a neighbor and put nine of the little porkers in a burlap sack and stuck it in the trunk of the car. Mike likes to go places with me, he follows me around all the time. Anyway, he sneaked into the back of the car and I didn't know he was there. Later, when I got in and started the car, the pigs all squealed at once setting up a terrible racket. Mark didn't know the pigs were there and was so frightened he couldn't talk for three days. Seems like he stuttered from then on.

Putting tongue in cheek, I labeled this Spasmophemia porcus.

Mark was a middle child. In addition to the older brother who excelled at whatever he tried (he was a star baseball pitcher, top student and successful newspaper carrier), there was a three-year-old sister, a precocious imp with puckish dimples and huge brown eyes. According to Mrs. Swenson, the sun rose and set in little Gigi.

the therapy employed

Working with young stutterers, especially within a school setting, is particularly challenging. It is sobering to note, then, that clinicians working in the schools report that their training was lacking or deficient with respect to therapy for this group of stutterers (Duncan, 1967). There are several unique problems involved in working with these children:

> Several thorny problems confront a public school speech therapist when working with young stutterers: (1) precipitating causes (factors which set the problem into motion) and maintaining agents (factors which keep the problem going once it has been started) may still be operating in the child's home and school situation. (2) Young children frequently lack the insight and cooperation necessary to analyze their problem rationally and objectively. (3) It is difficult for children to freely verbalize their internal feelings. (4) Children can confront themselves with unpleasant and feared experiences only with great difficulty; the desire to escape is very strong. (5) The speech therapist is identified in the child's mind with the teaching personnel who may be penalizing or disturbing listeners. In addition, the therapist may find himself identified with authority figures; this tends to be deleterious to the development of a therapeutic relationship. (6). The type of therapeutic program best suited for young

stutterers is often difficult to implement with the aegis of the public school. (Emerick, 1965, p. 398)

With the exception of a few recent excellent publications (Luper and Mulder, 1964; Speech Foundation of America, 1964; Cooper, 1965), the literature relative to this problem is sadly deficient.

It does not take one long to discover that adapting adult stuttering therapy to children is easier to write about than to do. Even the most resistant of adults will respond in some fashion, but Mark, as do many young stutterers, simply repeated "I don't know" or "beats me" to all my queries. Play therapy came to mind but, alas, descriptions of this approach tend to be rather vague and esoteric. There is little of practical value for the public school speech clinician in these writings. So, it was necessary to devise a goal oriented program combining what I hoped were the best aspects of play therapy and contemporary adult stuttering therapy. The therapy approach has been described elsewhere (Emerick, 1965), and I will only briefly review the major goals that guided my work with Mark:

Goal One—Associate speech with pleasure. We had to put the fun back into talking, and we did this by means of three subgoals: (1) Associate speaking with interpersonal sharing. Mark and I formed a speech club, he gave it a name, and we decided upon passwords and other verbal rituals. We built models of boats and airplanes, studying the instructions together —often aloud—and making decisions regarding the structuring and painting of the models. We caught and classified insects for Mark's collection. (2) Associate speaking with reward. At the beginning of each therapy session, I presented Mark with two clues. The first clue was to a hidden treasure (secreted in the room) and the second clue involved a secret word which, if uttered during the therapy session, would also yield a small reward. (3) Associate speaking with a feeling of adequacy. We used choral reading and simultaneous speaking, talking and reading with masking noise in our ears; we did some role playing with masks that we had made.

Goal Two—Ventilate the feelings and pressures. Since children seem to find it so difficult to experience verbal catharsis, it was necessary to employ alternate methods. Three subgoals were devised: (1) Play out the feelings. Mark drew pictures of things that made him afraid, angry or upset—and then destroyed the drawings. Clay was used for the same purpose. (2) Reduce the frustration of stuttering. Mark threw bean bags at the wall when he stuttered, and he pummelled a punching bag for each block he had. He collected quotas of stuttering to purchase token penalties for the clinician. (3) Act out the penalty and frustration associated with stuttering. Mark and I role-played situations that made him mad or afraid and situations in which he had been penalized for stuttering.

Goal Three—Take the pain out of stuttering. Mark was frustrated and bewildered by his problem, and he needed to learn that, even if he did stutter, he would not fall apart. Two subgoals were employed: (1) Associate stuttering with objectivity. I treated Mark's stuttering behavior as something interesting, something to study. We duplicated each other's stuttering, we made up new kinds and studied them in the mirror. We put on stethoscopes and listened intently to each other's stuttering. (2) Associate stuttering with reward. I have found that it is very difficult to get children to stutter on purpose as a direct goal. So, with Mark we did it indirectly by rewarding blocks with candy or giving him a chance to move in a game of checkers.

Goal Four—Make the mistakes more easily. The central theme in Mark's therapy program was learning to stutter in an easier, simpler fashion. This was accomplished in three subgoals: (1) Discovering how other people talk. Mark and I listened to tapes of stutterers and non-stutterers, trying to discover the ways in which people interrupt themselves. We made comparisons to Mark's stuttering. (2) Sharing and duplicating stuttering. When Mark blocked, I joined in matching my "stuttering" closely to his and then gradually shifting to an easier, smoother type of repetitious or prolonged stuttering. Mark helped me pull out of blocks. (3) Signal practice and a variety of easy stuttering. I stressed vivid comparison between hard and easy stuttering and had Mark shift from hard to easy and back to hard again as I raised and lowered my hand. We gave Navy commands to one another in duplicate, with one easy and one hard stuttering.

Goal Five—Associate fluency with communicative stress. It is not difficult for a stutterer to change his speech behavior in a clinic room with an empathic speech clinician. But the world is full of disturbing and distracting circumstances, and barriers must be built against hurry, competition, and listener disturbances. Three subgoals were employed: (1) Solving problems with speech. I presented Mark with a series of problems which he attempted to solve out loud; most of the problems were situations involving listener reactions to stuttering. (2) Resisting disturbing influences. Mark attempted to talk while I introduced distracting influences, such as looking away, grimacing, interrupting, etc. (3) Doing real life situations. Mark and I went out to stores and on house-to-house surveys to practice things that we had learned in the Clinic.

Mark was seen three days a week for hour sessions, and, even though the therapy sessions were held after school, he looked forward to the meetings. In addition, I saw Mrs. Swenson once weekly as part of a counseling and education program.

results and follow-up

After a somewhat slow and uncertain start during which Mark tested my motives and purposes, he made a startlingly swift recovery. Initially, he appeared to assume that I, like most other people who had tried to help him, wanted him to stop or hide stuttering. Slowly—it took at least six weeks—he began to realize that we were doing battle with a common enemy and that what we were after was changing the way he stuttered, not inhibiting it. Mark was brought to the Clinic in January and by late spring he was talking more, talking more easily and definitely enjoying it. He was sliding out of even his worst blocks in almost all speaking situations. His parents and his teacher reported that, after an initial period of acting out (expressions of hostility and aggression toward his classmates and siblings), Mark seemed happier and less withdrawn. I was dubious, however, of this rapid recovery and so he was enrolled in an intensive summer group therapy program (the children were seen daily for an hour) with three children about his age. By the end of the second week, Mark had taken over leadership of this group. It was delightful. I sat back and watched Mark move through the goals and subgoals with the group even as we had done that spring. Not only did he do a magnificent job of therapy, he stabilized his own progress to boot!

The parents also changed dramatically, but, and I feel that this is significant, only after Mark's speech began to improve. This has been repeated a number of times in my clinical experience with parents of young stutterers; they appear to become much more amenable to counseling and therapeutic suggestions when they see some results with their child. At any rate that's what happened with Mark's father. He was impressed by the rapid change in his son's speech (he later confided that he had harbored deep feelings of futility and doubt in bringing Mark for speech help), and he was even more impressed with the clinician's relationship with his son. Mark came home from our adventures bubbling over with what he and his speech therapist had done; I'm afraid he made me sound like a combination of Mark Twain, Henry David Thoreau and Charles Atlas. Yet, apparently this propelled Mr. Swenson to re-evaluate his relationship with his son. He let his assistant manager take over the restaurant and went fishing with his son; they took a canoe trip down the river; and, yes, they even collected bugs! To his surprise, Mr. Swenson found that he enjoyed the nature study with his son, and when last I heard, they both had joined the local Audubon Society. Mrs. Swenson became my most enchanted parent. She was able to see what her own speech and her emphasis on good speech was doing to Mark, and she modified her behavior consonant with my suggestions. She sang the Clinic's praises up and down the region, she spread the gospel of stuttering according to Emerick to other parents, and she even sent us several speech correction majors from the high school!

Mark was followed up for four years after his dismissal from the Clinic. When I left the area to assume my present position, he was in the sixth grade and was doing well with respect to both speech and academics. I interviewed his teacher, a dynamic young gal who was new to the school system, not long before we moved from the town. She informed me rather firmly that Mark was, in her opinion, a normal speaker, that his parents considered him a normal speaker, and that Mark considered himself a normal speaker. Then she added didactically, "Oh, yes, I did read in Mark's cumulative folder that he had gone through a period of stuttering. But then, don't all children?" I nodded sagely, closed my briefcase and silently crept away.

comments and interpretation

As I reviewed my files in preparation for this writing, again I was amazed at the swiftness and completeness of Mark's recovery from stuttering. The question is: Why? What did I do to cut through so rapidly all the negative reinforcement and mismanagement he had endured at the hands of his parents and his peers? Did Mark recover in spite of what I did instead of because of it? Did I appear on the scene at just the right time? Was Mark ready to recover and I just a catalyst? Could any warm, supportive person have done the same things? In other words, what was my relationship to the therapeutic success? What therapeutic roles did I play and how did I portray them? How important was I to the therapy process? What were the key elements in this instance of successful therapy? After carefully reviewing the clinical data and reliving the therapeutic experience—as well as engaging in agonizingly prolonged contemplation—the following items emerged as the crucial determinants in Mark's successful rehabilitation:

1. Mark needed to identify with a male figure, and I was able to fulfill for him the role of father or big brother. This was perhaps the most important aspect of the therapy experience; indeed, solely by this positive bond with the clinician—which developed very rapidly from the first meeting—I feel that his stuttering problem would have been at least partly solved. There were several interesting and rather unique facets involved in Mark's identification with the clinician. The first aspect, and most probably the basis for the rapidity with which the relationship developed, was that we shared a mutual interest in the out-of-doors. We had an instant basis for communication since I am an amateur naturalist, hunter and fisherman. This leads to the second facet. The interests we shared could be enjoyed without verbal communication. Mark seemed to want deeply to just follow someone around, to do things with someone without talking, to just share and relate on a nonverbal level. As a stutterer, I well remember the importance of this in my own life. My grandfather, a taciturn old Cousin Jack copper miner from the Upper Peninsula of Michigan, provided an island of silent safety in a frightening verbal world. Although he never would have admitted it and indeed dismissed all modern notions about child rearing as so much bloody balderdash (his language was more colorful), he seemed to sense what a little kid hurt in the mouth needed. We did many timeless and simple things together quietly, but most of all I remember the silent ritual performed each evening behind his cabin in the northwoods. Sitting side by side on a crude bench he had made with his own hands, we watched the sun slowly make its descent behind the trees and wash the pines with fingers of 'pale gold. He neither tolerated or desired chatter, and all others were banished from this evening rite. Perhaps, Mark's parents did not understand—at least at first—the silent hikes along the river, the quiet fishing trips, but Grandfather would have understood and approved.

Grandfather would have also approved of the third facet of the identification between Mark and myself for he loathed sham or facade. I found that I really liked the kid and enjoyed doing things with him, and I think he realized this very soon. We did many extra things together that we both enjoyed: we built models of birds and painted them; I taught Mark how to shoot a bow and arrow; and Mark taught me how to collect and classify insects. Why did I do all this? Perhaps because Mark reminded me so vividly of my own "ghosts of stuttering past," of the bewildered and belligerent second grader that I had been. Interestingly, because of the intense identification and extensive interaction, Mark was forced to drop his defenses. When one is with another person for such prolonged intervals of time, one cannot keep from revealing his real self. Thus, not only were we then able to confront the stuttering problem directly, but also Mark had the vivid experience of acceptance of his real self from another human being.

Specifically, how did I portray the role of father or big brother? Actually, it was an evolving role. At first I was good old Dad in a wool shirt, warm and friendly, trustworthy and smelling of pipe smoke and old leathers, sharing blocks and relating closely by nonverbal means. As Mark's speech improved and he derived satisfaction from this, and as his own father began to take over his heretofore abrogated role, I gradually withdrew and became a somewhat aloof patrician sort of pater, directing behavior by precept but not as intimately involved.

2. Mark desperately needed to share his stuttering problem with another human being, and I fulfilled this need—apparently at the right time. He was, as I indicated above, bewildered and frustrated with the intermittent speech barriers. He seemed to feel that he was the only one in the world with this strange speech disturbance. No one mentioned stuttering except to tell him occasionally to try harder to stop it, and he knew he could not for the more he tried, the worse it became. Then suddenly he was confronted with someone who not only talked a lot about stuttering and was interested in it but, even more astoundingly, was willing to stutter along with him, sharing the frustrating fixations and the dreadful tremors that seemed to run away with his mouth.

Initially, Mark was very cautious about sharing his stuttering with the clinician. He had to be sure that I could be trusted, that I would not suddenly laugh at his blocks or in some manner reveal disapproval. Gradually, he tested me with some of his most severe stuttering and found that, rather than rejection, pity or humor, it was met with curiosity and genuine interest. Then, augmented by the nonverbal identification described above, a true meeting of one human being with another emerged; the I-thou relationship discussed by Backus (1960) burgeoned forth in full flower. It is one thing to stand apart and tell a young boy that there is nothing to fear in the dark alley of his stuttering, but it is another thing to go through the alley with him.

In summary, sharing was a very crucial aspect in this successful therapy experience. My role of "Sharer" was characterized initially by an active participation in Mark's problem, an intense inter-personal commonality and feeling of comradeship between Mark and myself. We were going into the fight together to do battle with stuttering. A frequent phenomenon of intensive group interaction is the tendency for the members to turn inward, directing all their communication to and deriving all their satisfaction from individuals going through the common experience. Despite the potential dangers (mainly the tendency to form a safe stuttering society to the exclusion of real life adjustments) involved, it is my impression that stutterers and their clinicians need to form this intensive sort of group feeling during the initial stages of therapy. It serves to make their stuttering problem legitimate within a special social setting. Gradually, I withdrew from such active sharing with Mark and became by stages a rather passive observer. As he assumed more responsibility for his own behavior, I ceased to monitor moments of stuttering with him and merely rewarded his efforts as an interested spectator. The gradual disengagement of the therapist from the client is a basic element in stuttering therapy. Initially, the stutterers appear to need to lean rather heavily upon the clinician, but they can and must learn to support their own weight.

3. I was able to stand the uncertainty of the first few weeks of therapy. Mark was not like an adult stutterer; he did not provide me with much feedback or even an active resistance to therapy. Passive resistance is the young stutterers' forte. It is easy to understand why some clinicians, especially those who are attuned to "doing things" in therapy (and who grow forgetful that not all behavior is rationally determined) become impatient and exasperated with young stutterers. Sometimes the clinician gives up in despair. Children are all too aware when this occurs. I worked with one boy who whispered to me on the first day that the last "speech teacher" had told his mother that nothing could be done with his stuttering for a long time. He tested me for three months before he was convinced that I was not going to give up.

Though Mark related well to me on a nonverbal level, it was at least six weeks before we could openly deal with stuttering on the level described in the goals and subgoals delineated above. My contribution to successful therapy during this testing period was, I believe, the absence of any overt reactions to his lack of responsiveness.

4. Another important factor in the successful termination of therapy with Mark was the honesty of the clinical relationship (Cooper, 1965). It is obvious that identification, sharing and honesty are interrelated. It was necessary with the intense identification that emerged, with the prolonged interpersonal contact and the

sense of sharing that developed, that Mark would be forced to be honest with the clinician.

I attempted, by way of example, to be scrupulously honest with Mark. First, I was honest about his stuttering. Instead of pretending that it didn't exist, I acknowledged that he was having some difficulty and that we would see what we could do to make it easier to talk. No false reassurance, no superficial glossing over of the problem. Secondly, since I was seeing his parents, I was honest with Mark about this. I asked Mark's permission to talk with his parents regarding some of the things we were doing in therapy. I recorded my interviews with Mrs. Swenson and Mark was permitted to listen to these; he made up check lists of the things his parents were supposed to be doing and devised a report card for them. The parents knew that Mark was doing this, and he knew that they knew. This had quite an impact upon him. One day when we were using Indian talk to identify the cues associated with non-stuttered speech, he said: "You not talk with forked tongue, you talk true."

5. I was able to inspire confidence in the clinician and engender excitement and enthusiasm for the therapy program. Some clinicians, especially those who have had limited experience working with stutterers during their training, are fearful of stuttering therapy. They are anxious lest they do something to make the problem worse. Hence, in reality, they are afraid of the disorder of stuttering. They tend to be timid and temporizing in their approach; they cannot inspire confidence for their own anxieties show through.

Why was I able to obtain Mark's commitment to the therapist and the therapy? There are several reasons. First, this was a new adventure for me too, and my own enthusiasm and excitement as I bayed along the trail may have been infectious. Perhaps we were both drawn into an experience not unlike the familiar Hawthorne effect. Was I more "natural" because this was the first time that I had explored the goals with a young stutterer? It seemed that way. In a sense, then, I was fulfilling the role of explorer and Mark was caught up in the adventure into unknown lands. In the second place, even though the procedures I employed were relatively new for me, at least as they applied to the young stutterer, I was convinced that they would work. I expected him to improve for I knew that the therapy was based upon solid theoretical and clinical evidence. Finally, and perhaps most important, my therapeutic approach flows from a philosophy of life that encompasses a commitment to the principle of performing everything I do at the limit of my capacity. I decided long ago that I would rather wear out than rust out.

So, with Mark there was an element of suggestion, but I frankly see nothing wrong with this much maligned element in *all* therapy if it is used judiciously and (a) is designed to get the stutterer "hooked" on the therapy approach, (b) is based upon some creditable rationale, and (c) is not the sole basis for therapy. In Mark's eyes, therefore, at least during the first part of the therapy program, I played the role of healer. This healer, as I think he viewed it, was first a magic sorcerer whose priestly presence was sufficient to give surcease. Then, as we worked together, and Mark began to assume some responsibility for his therapy, we became like a surgical team with my role that of experienced surgeon guiding the hands of the young intern. Later, he became his own healer coming to me only now and then for suggestions.

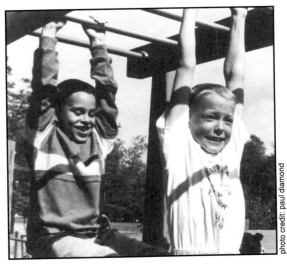

photo credit: paul diamond

A CLINICAL FAILURE: SHERRIE
CLINICIAN: LON EMERICK

Confronting one's failures is far more difficult than scrutinizing clinical success but is probably more instructive. It certainly is more sobering. It is easy to blame the schools (how can you do stuttering therapy in the public schools), the parents (how can you help a child with parents like that?) or the child himself (he just wasn't motivated to change the way he talked). Whenever I get to feeling over-confident as a clinician, I sit in my study chambers and parade my therapy failures past until I can see the very whites of their eyes. My room becomes an I. A. C. booth and at 120 dB the stut- terers are crying out: "When I resisted you tried not to understand," "When I struggled you shared not my tremors," "When I needed intensive help you were writing memos and filling out requisitions." And the loudest voice of all, because it is a silent one, is that of Sherrie.

Sherrie came to the Clinic less than a month after Mark was seen for initial appraisal. Her mother, Mrs. Ford, after hearing me discuss the problem of stuttering at a child study group, pleaded with me to evaluate and work with her child. Since Sherrie had re- cently been seen for therapy in the school, I first contacted the speech clinician. Miss Hamre indicated that Sherrie had been re- leased from her caseload because, in her view, there was nothing that could be done with her until she was older and more amenable to therapy. She added, "I can't seem to do a thing with Sherrie, she just sits there when we go through her speech workbook and says 'I don't know' to every question I ask. I don't think young stutterers can be worked with until they reach some level of reasoning, do you? Well, anyway, I would sure like to have you see her and, say, could I come over and observe?" Before the date arranged for the evalua- tion, however, Miss Hatten, principal of the elementary school which Sherrie attended, called and demanded to see me forthwith. A stere- otyped and hopefully almost extinct school marm, with wedge heels, blue hair pulled back in a bun and frameless spectacles, she insisted that the child's problem be solved within the aegis of the school. "We can handle our problems here, thank you," she said primly with tensed platysma muscles. I assured Miss Hatten that I merely meant to help and that both the mother and the speech therapist wanted to have the child seen in the Clinic. Reluctantly, with some clucking and posturing, she conceded to implement the referral. At last I got to see Sherrie.

I shall never forget the little gal, a small eight year old with a pretty oval face, framed with honey-brown hair and punctuated by eyes bluer than Lake Superior on an October morning. She liked ice cream, hated spinach and giggled like other eight-year-old girls. But she didn't giggle much; she was stuttering quite severely. She appeared to go into a trance when she stuttered: she fixated on an articulatory posture, her eyes turned upward slightly and glazed and her whole body became rigid. Finally, after a silent impasse for from five to ten seconds, she either blurted out the word or gave up the speech attempt. Although she seemed to have no sound, word or situation fears, her moments of stuttering were quite consistent in their loci (Bloodstein, 1960). After release from the block, she spoke fluently for perhaps ten to fifteen words as if looking back and saying, "I don't know what was going on there but it really was not me, see me talk fluently." Stuttering for her—when I asked her to draw what represented her stuttering (Sheehan, 1962)—was a tiny bird on a cold mid-winter night beating feebly and futilely upon a picture window. Inside was a family, all warm and cozy, but the sparrow could not join them through the barrier even though she could see them so clearly. Bewildered and frightened by her stuttering, Sherrie was very much like the little sparrow she drew. One time during the first few weeks of therapy we were playing with a tape recorder, and she wanted to hear her own speech. When she heard the blocks, which apparently she had never heard quite so vividly before, she climbed up in my lap and wept softly for the rest of the hour.

The onset of stuttering was lost in the dim passages of her parents' memories. Neither father nor mother could recall when Sherrie first began to have difficulty with speech. Mrs. Ford said that it seemed as if the child had always stuttered. She did remember, however, that when Sherrie was about four years old, a relative had suggested a remedy for the stuttering problem. The "cure" consisted of a bottle of mineral oil and an eyedropper to be used as follows: whenever Sherrie blocked, Mrs. Ford was to squirt an eyedropper full of oil down the child's throat. I wonder if Skinner would term that an aversive stimulus? Sherrie's problem had grown steadily worse (despite the lube job) and the stuttering behavior was now more ubiquitous than it had ever been. Mrs. Ford felt that Sherrie was a very sensitive child because she became upset with changes in her environment, such as an overnight guest who altered the sleeping arrangements, any deviation from household routine and so forth. Sherrie was seen by a clinical psychologist at a Child Guidance Clinic; his report said that she obtained an I.Q. of 136 on the WISC, that the results of projective testing revealed nothing of significance, and that she stuttered.

Sherrie's mother was an attractive woman in her late thirties who had raised three children to school age and then returned to college in order to complete her degree in language and literature.

When I first met her, she was in her senior year and eagerly looking forward to a career as a high school teacher. Mrs. Ford talked at great length about the things she had done for Sherrie, the sacrifices she had made and all the advantages that would accrue to her daughter and her family with two salaries to support the family. However, she appeared to do little *with* her children, especially Sherrie. The topic of stuttering was taboo in the household. Despite the fact that Sherrie had been seen for therapy by a public school clinician, no one, not even Mrs. Ford, acknowledged that talking was sometimes a tough job. Each time that Sherrie stuttered, the family members reacted as a unit: despite the obvious struggles, regardless of the tonic postures, everyone pretended that her difficulty did not even exist. This elaborate code of silence made matters worse for not only did Sherrie have bewildering speech barriers, but she felt it was also something dreadful and unspeakable. Mrs. Ford had little faith that speech therapy would really help her daughter, but she wanted to take every opportunity to obtain professional assistance. "I must do everything I can for her," she often told me. She talked of predestination and appeared to hold the view that someday Sherrie would simply wake up and be free of the stuttering problem. The theme that ran through the counseling sessions with Mrs. Ford was embarrassment; she viewed Sherrie's stuttering problem as an outward and visible sign by which others could impugn her effectiveness as a mother.

Mr. Ford, who at 52 was thirteen years older than his wife, edited and published a small town weekly newspaper, a position he had held for over 20 years. Despite this enormous drain on his time, he was attempting to write the Great American Novel during minutes stolen from his newspaper—and from his family. He was a gentle, blinking, tweedy, distracted sort of man, in the world but not of it. Surprised to find himself married, he was overwhelmed in a bemused sort of way to have sired three children. He indicated that raising the children was his wife's responsibility—he was much too busy with the paper and with his novel. When I pressed him he just shrugged, said that he had stuttered as a youth and had grown out of it. No doubt Sherrie inherited the tendency, he observed, but he was sure that she too would grow out of it. "Children's maturation is a series of phases," he said finally, "and this is merely another phase." Because Mr. Ford was so much like Elwood Dowd in my well-thumbed copy of the play *Harvey* by Mary Chase, perhaps I did not seriously try to change him.

Sherrie was the youngest of three children. She had a twelve-year-old brother in the sixth grade and a sister of fourteen in the eighth grade. Both of these children had normal speech and were doing exceptionally well in school. They furthermore shared the same interests and were very close, tending to form a dyad which excluded their little sister.

the therapy employed

I attempted to employ basically the same type of therapy that guided my approach with Mark although I recognized that one can never step in the same therapy room twice, nor is the clinician or the client the same. At any rate, the goals as delineated in the presentation of a successful therapy experience (see A Clinical Success: Mark) were utilized as I met with Sherrie two hours a week. However, we never did make much forward progress relative to the goals and subgoals; most of the therapy time was spent trying to find some basis for relating to the child. Establishing rapport was the hangup that I never was able to solve.

results and follow-up

Despite what I felt were my best efforts, I never did break through to Sherrie. She seemed to want to relate to me, to let me know and share the agony that was her stuttering, but I could not find the right key to let her out of her protective shell. Although she never said it, her whole manner cried out, "You want me to stop stuttering like those other people, my teachers and that speech person. But it's too frightening to change. I can't do it. If I just keep quiet, if I shrink inward, this too shall pass away." And so like a startled little fawn, she remained frozen and inert. As I introduced each goal there was a faint flicker of enthusiasm, perhaps even a little crack in her marble composure; but then, as if tricked, she retreated to her shell.

After working with her all spring (from March until the end of May) with no success, I decided to enroll Sherrie in an intensive summer program of group therapy for young stutterers. Perhaps her peers could do what I could not. However, Sherrie quickly became the isolate of the group. She sat silently as the others worked upon the various goals. At first the children directed a lot of attention to her in an attempt to bring her into the fold. But her resistance continued and the young stutterers isolated her from interaction. Her mother removed Sherrie from therapy at midpoint of the summer program, explaining it was time for their vacation. The truth was probably closer to the fact that Sherrie was doing some acting out at home. She was being very hostile, tearing up some of her siblings' prized possessions, tormenting the family dog and taking out some of her aggression on herself in the form of headbanging. Mrs. Ford felt that therapy was upsetting her daughter because she certainly wasn't acting like her sweet little self. "And her speech seemed to be getting worse, too," Mrs. Ford added.

Despite my pleas that these might be good signs, that things sometimes get worse before they get better, therapy was terminated

Sherrie was followed up for three years. After the unsuccessful half-summer of speech therapy, Mrs. Ford took the child to a pediatrician who recommended a prolonged course of tranquilizers; the mother reported these had little meliorative effect. When the family was last contacted, the problem appeared to have taken on some grave dimensions. Sherrie was still stuttering badly. She was also manifesting masochistic behavior, pinching herself, headbanging and pulling out her eye lashes. A child psychiatrist was working with her.

comments and interpretations

Why did I fail with Sherrie? The family problems were obvious, but why was I impotent in the face of them? Should I, could I, have persuaded Mrs. Ford to leave Sherrie in the group therapy? What had I done—or not done—that led to such abject failure? From my point of view there are some hard-won answers to these questions. Are they rationalizations? Perhaps the reader can judge better than I.

1. The central factor in my therapeutic failure with Sherrie was that I did not maintain a professionally objective attitude in my relationship with her. More simply, I blew my therapeutic cool. There seems to be a line like a razor's edge between a solid empathic relationship and emotional involvement with a client. I cared too much but not well.

Why did this occur? Why did I want to "protect" Sherrie rather than work with her? After prolonged and careful consideration, there seem to be two basic reasons for my loss of objectivity. First, I tend to have a rather intense affinity for and ready emotional attachment to little girls. Second and more important in the case of Sherrie, I believe that my concern for her, my subjective feelings regarding the complexity and severity of her stuttering must have shown through to her. Did she sense my anxiety and sometimes my panic in the face of her problem? Rather than helping her do battle with the stuttering, I am afraid that emotionally I only wanted to shield her from it. Thus, I became her protector to the exclusion of any other role. I wanted, it would seem, not to provide clinical assistance but a sanctuary for the troubled sparrow. This is not an uncommon occurrence in the helping professions, especially among those who work with severely handicapped children, the deaf, mentally retarded and so forth. Instend of pushing them to achieve what they could achieve, in many instances, the workers protect and buffer the children because they have already suffered so much at the hands of fate.

I further compounded my error with Sherrie because I responded to her resistance to therapy not rationally but emotionally. Redoubling my efforts I attempted to storm her defenses too rapidly and thus frightened her even further.

2. My negative expectations regarding the outcome of therapy were unwittingly communicated to Sherrie. I am convinced that what the clinician thinks the client can do, that shall he do; in other words, after Parkinson, the client's behavior expands to fit the clinician's concept of his potential. Let me illustrate this with an anecdote that arose in our practice with adult aphasics in a Veterans' Hospital:

> An advanced graduate student, an excellent clinician, was working for the first time with an adult aphasic. I had done the original examination on the patient and had also had several sessions with him but wanted the student to work with the patient and make her own assessment of the patient's prognosis. She presented the aphasic with several picture cards and requested that he name them. The patient looked at her and said something that sounded to her ears like "I know, I know," in an exasperated tone. The student responded firmly: "I know you know, Mr. Tolonen, now try these words in a short phrase." Damned if he didn't, and I nearly fell off the chair. For you see, the patient's first name was Heino (pronounced I know), and, heretofore, he had simply repeated his name to each request for verbalization!

I felt that the prognosis for Sherrie was poor on the basis of the family patterns, her detachment from her stuttering behavior and the first unsuccessful therapy experiences. But there was another and perhaps more important reason for making a doleful prediction: I have a poor therapy record with female stutterers. I have been able to substantially help not more than one or two out of the dozen or so that have come to me for therapy. Do we condition our *own* behavior when we make a prognosis? Does this communicate to the client on some level? I think it did with Sherrie.

3. A third factor contributing to the unsuccessful therapy experience with Sherrie was the difficulty in obtaining positive identification with the clinician. To some extent this may have been a sex barrier since we could not share the masculine activities as I had done with Mark and the other young stutterers. Having no sister, and no children at the time, I felt that all little girls are made of sugar and spice and everything nice. Perhaps Sherrie, too, would have responded to a fishing trip or a hike along the river in search of fossils. Subsequently, we have experimented with men and women student clinicians for female stutterers; we seem to get the best results by employing a male-female team which appears to comprise a "therapeutic family." In my view, identification with the

clinician is the crucial factor in therapeutic success with stutterers of all ages. It provides, as it were, a basis for engendering movement of the client in terms of the specific speech goals. Although negative identification is sometimes useful when working with adult stutterers ("I am going to show that son-of-a-gun that I can do it!"), it doesn't seem to be too helpful in our work with the young stutterers. Most of the discussion in this paper has dealt with assumed roles, that is, "parts" that the clinician portrayed as a volitional aspect of his therapeutic armamentarium. But there are also ascribed roles, roles that are assigned by the stutterer for the clinician to play. Despite my efforts to obtain positive identification as an ally, despite my attempts to share the stuttering problem with Sherrie, she saw me solely in the role of magic healer. She seemed to sit in the therapy session in tense expectation that somehow I would take away the stuttering; at times, frightened little bird that she was, she even appeared to furtively reach out to touch the robe.

4. With Sherrie, I committed a very common error in the clinical management of stuttering: I failed to consider fully the differences among stutterers. I stand guilty of trying to treat the problem of stuttering, not the person who stutters. There is a growing realization that one has not said much that is definitive about the individual by simply designating his problem as stuttering (Robinson, 1965). Impressed by the response of Mark to the therapy regimen, it appears that I applied the goals without considering the special needs that Sherrie presented. Unable to understand exactly what she needed and wanted from me, I applied what I felt was the best possible remediation. We need to know much more about differences *among* stutterers.

5. It is with some reluctance that I include this remaining factor in my therapeutic failure with Sherrie. But it is one that all of us face and I must report it. I simply could not or did not take the time necessary to make the breakthrough to Sherrie. One cannot be all things to all stutterers even though he may desperately want to be; there are memos to write, clinics to plan, reports to file and other cases that hunger for services. I was able to see Sherrie only twice weekly—at least I felt so at the time. Perhaps I could have done the job with a more intensive approach. Of all the sad things of therapy with stutterers, the saddest is this: it might have been with Sherrie.

references

Backus, O., "The Study of Psychological Processes in Speech Therapists," In Barbara, D. (ed) *Psychological and Psychiatric Aspects to Speech and Hearing*, 1960, C. C. Thomas.

Bloodstein, O., "The Development of Stuttering: 1. Changes in Nine Basic Features," *Journal of Speech and Hearing Disorders, 25,* 1960, pp. 219-237.

Cooper, E., "Structuring Therapy for Therapist and Stuttering Child," *Journal of Speech and Hearing Disorders, 30,* 1965, pp. 75-78.

Cooper, E., "An Inquiry into the Use of Inter-personal Communication as a Source of Therapy With Stutterers," In D. Barbara, (ed) *New Directions in Stuttering,* Springfield: C. C. Thomas, 1965.

Duncan, R., "A Survey of Academic and Clinical Training of Public School Speech Clinicians in the Area of Stuttering," Unpublished Master's Thesis, Michigan State University, 1967.

Emerck, L., "Therapy for Young Stutterers," *Exceptional Children, 31,* 1965, pp. 398-402.

Emerick, L., and Teigland, A., "Pediatricians and Speech Disorders," *Central States Speech Journal, 26,* 1965, pp. 290-294.

Fraser, M. (publisher), *Treatment of the Young Stutterer in the School,* Memphis, Tennessee: Speech Foundation of America, Publication No. 4, 1964.

Luper, H. and Mulder, R., *Stuttering: Therapy for Children.* Englewood Cliffs: Prentice-Hall, Inc., 1964.

Robinson, F., *An Introduction to Stuttering.* Englewood Cliffs: Prentice-Hall, Inc., 1964, pp. 77.

Sheehan, J., Cortese, P. and Hadley, R., "Guilt, Shame, and Tension in Graphic Projections of Stuttering," *Journal of Speech and Hearing Disorders, 27,* 1962, pp. 129-139.

Van Riper, C., *Speech Correction: Principles and Methods.* Englewood Cliffs: Prentice-Hall, Inc., 1963.

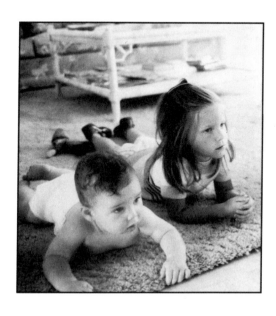

A CLINICAL SUCCESS: CORA
CLINICIAN: HUGO GREGORY

Cora was a 23-year-old Negro female of large build, semi-neatly groomed and with the potential of being an attractive person. She was employed by a stock broker as an editor of consultation reports. Her ambition was to be a teacher. She holds a B.A. degree in English.

The history revealed that she had grown up in Alabama. At age 2 she was sent to live with her maternal grandparents. The parents, according to Cora, were having difficulty and wanted "to get rid of the product of their union." She had no relationship with her parents. The subject reported that her grandfather was a loving person, but that her grandmother resented the fact that "I represented the dream of what she had put into her last child." Our initial impression of Cora was that she was distant and somewhat angry toward her family, her employer, men, and the environment in which she had been reared. She described herself as growing up alone. Our earliest impression was that to do something successful with a group meant a great deal to her, but she had a very high estimation of what was "success." "Success" probably meant being "the best." She verbalized her resentment that the environment in which she was reared was not as perfect as it should be.

Cora was a moderately severe stutterer. She manifested some severely tonic blocks, especially on bilabial sounds, that lasted as long as seven seconds. Articulation was slurred, and she rambled as she spoke—both characteristics were thought to be secondary manifestations of stuttering. She blocked on most of the consonant sounds and often on medial and final syllables. There were contortions of the face, squinting of the eyes, and very poor eye contact. Her eyes would water as she spoke. During speech she said her head "was hot." In summary, Cora was very anxious and tense as she spoke.

The client related that the grandmother recalled that she began stuttering at 9 years of age when Cora entered "a new room at school."

Cora was seen one hour a week in individual therapy and two hours a week in group therapy for 9 months. Therapy began with a case history. During these discussion oriented interviews, the clinician's objective was to establish an atmosphere in which the client would feel that we were interested in her as a person and wanted to understand her problem as well as we could. Such questions were discussed as the following: What do you think cause your problem? What have you been told will help stutterers? What have you done for your stuttering?

The same topics were pursued in the group sessions in which there were nine other stutterers. The clinician rewarded the clients' contributions by repeating them at the beginning of subsequent sessions or by asking them to share a certain observation with the others in the group.

Cora expressed the opinion that many people believe stuttering is associated with a lack of intelligence—that when the stutterer gets stuck or substitutes a word, it is due to a limited vocabulary. This revealed something about Cora's concept pertaining to listeners' reactions as contrasted with other stutterers who report people telling them that stutterers are more intelligent—that they think faster than they speak or that they must have a large vocabulary to substitute so frequently. Other information of this type came out; and after hearing herself on the tape recorder at the second session, she said, "I sound much more literate and don't block nearly as long as I thought."

The emerging picture of her self-concept was interesting. She had a "superior" manner in a way, very high standards for herself, and felt that she never quite measured up as she should. This was interpreted as a compensation for the way she felt about her background of being reared in a low socio-economic environment and of being rejected by her parents and grandmother.

I think it was very important for this client to find in therapy an opportunity to explore her feelings about her previous life experiences. I was the group clinician, and, fortunately, her therapist in individual sessions was a person who could listen well and offer appropriate comments which reinforced her thoughtful statements. Her clinician was also effective in providing interpretations which did not frighten the client during the early stages of therapy.

She revealed that she had undergone psychotherapy for three months, two years before. Testing done at that time showed that she was capable and had aptitude scores that coincided with people in the fields of English and philosophy. Cora said she was learning to "accept some things" about herself and that she was beginning to see that she "should not feel sorry for herself." Although she did not continue this counselling, it seemed to us that she had gained from this experience by being reassured about her ability and by being directed to an appraisal of her self-evaluations.

Following a discussion of the possible ways in which stuttering develops and the development of secondary symptoms, the client and the clinician worked together in analyzing and labelling the client's stuttering behavior. Mirror work and tape recordings were used in this process. Negative practive (imitating actual secondary manifestations) was used in the individual sessions. Cora began to realize what she was doing when she interrupted the speech flow or "stuttered." For example, she observed what she called a "double stuttering block" in which the tension would begin at one place of articulation and spread to another. The clinician was careful to give her support during this phase of therapy. She was told that she should expect to feel a little more anxious at this time in therapy and that actually her stuttering might seem somewhat worse as she forced herself to face it rather than concealing it as previously. The clinicians rewarded all of the clients for being willing to go ahead and talk regardless of their difficulty, and most especially they were rewarded for analyzing their speech behavior. Gradually, the idea was getting through to Cora that stuttering wasn't something that just happened, but it was the exaggerated pursing of the mouth, the dialating of the nostrils, the tensing of the jaw, etc., that she did when she talked. Furthermore, in doing the negative practice, the client began to see that she could modify and change the stuttering pattern.

Note: Oftentimes at this stage of therapy in which the direct modification work is being initiated, clinicians report that they have difficulty maintaining a balance between the more didactic approach to speech modification and the more understanding, permissive interview relationship which is important in changing attitude. In working with Cora, our objective was to establish the attitude of a cooperative effort between the clinician and the client. Thus, even in direct speech work considerable responsibility for analysis and modification should remain with the client. We tried to develop the idea of the clinician as a guide.

The subject was taught relaxation procedures using Jacobson's progressive and differential method.

She was given the following rationale:

1. In order to relieve the tension which you have observed in the speech mechanism, you must learn to be aware of the state of tension in the small and large muscle groups throughout the body.

2. Thinking of and striving for increased relaxation when under stress will provide a competing response which will help you be more calm.

She was encouraged to compare the tense and relaxed state of her arm during the relaxation exercise with the tense and less tense condition of her lips during speech. She was shown other ways that she could modify her speech response—voluntary stuttering (bounce, slide). Clinicians in the program used voluntary stuttering and Cora teased her clinician about using the "uh" vowel after every consonant such as saying " bu bu bu" in "busy."

As work progressed on speech modifications, the clinician provided leads and opportunities for the client to explore her attitudes and feelings. A more hopeful attitude toward being able to change her speech seemed to result in Cora being less anxious and tense at this time when speaking, and perhaps less anxious generally. She seemed to recognize, however, that she needed to spend clinical time exploring her attitudes and feelings toward herself and others.

Cora felt that her immediate supervisor where she worked was very perfectionistic. She said she avoided him "because he has admiration for articulate people and is intolerant of imperfection." This reference led to a more thorough consideration of the roots of her perfectionistic attitude. She expressed the idea that her perfectionistic attitude was related to her hostile feelings toward her family whom she saw as being so imperfect. As a direct result of these conversations, Cora decided on a course of action which included telling her supervisor about the stuttering program.

Cora's eye contact was much improved at this time and she was using voluntary stuttering in situations outside the clinic. When using the bounce pattern, she often went out of control on the second bounce. She said this happened because she was fearful of the listener's impatience. The clinician discussed the possibility that she was projecting her own impatience and perfection into the listener. At this time (the end of three months of therapy), Cora was beginning to use many new verbal labels, e.g., "projection," "rationalization," and "inferior feelings." She was exploring some interesting thoughts such as: "I felt incompetent and unequal and stuttering became the whipping boy of all the feelings of inadequacy," "I have never known a person who was perfect."

She labelled as rationalization her refusals to go to meetings of her college alumni organization because "I don't like the way the organization is run." She went to one meeting and had so much trouble introducing herself that she never returned.

Cora seemed to begin making discriminations concerning attitudes learned as a child and generalized to adulthood ("I'm surprised a grownup can be so fearful."). She was talking more to friends about her attitudes and this was interpreted as a generalization of behavior learned in the clinic. Friends told her she was much too serious and sensitive.

Cora was feeling increasingly good about her new speech pattern as she used cancellations, pull-outs, and new preparatory sets. She worked on phrasing, increased oral activity (she had a tendency not to open her mouth sufficiently, resulting in slurred speech), inflection, etc. She reported the changed speech pattern was beginning to come naturally. In talking with a male friend about her stuttering and the reason why she would not go into teaching, she found this friend was not "impressed" by her stuttering problem and did not see why it should prevent her from being a teacher.

In the group, she shared these thoughts and experiences freely and became admired by the others. This was very important reinforcement.

She reported enjoying humor and small talk with other women at work. For example, she had a "small talk" conversation with one woman at a coffee machine and this person came to talk with the client two more times that day.

The sessions during the last month of therapy were directed toward working out a plan for Cora to be her own therapist. In the group she said, "I plan to enter each speaking situation with techniques I've learned at the clinic, and, hopefully, they will become habit. I plan to continually evaluate performance." Her motto was "you experience, you reflect, you evaluate, and you change."

Shortly after leaving therapy, Cora took a position teaching English in an industrial training school. She thought this would be good for her as the students there would not be as great a challenge as those students in a regular academic program. She succeeded in the industrial school, and, one year later, she was appointed to a position in a large city school district.

At our last "reunion meeting," Cora appeared thrilled and happy with her present life situation. Her communication was very pleasant and adequate. The few stuttering blocks which she had were very mild and of a nature that would probably not be observed by a listener not aware that she had had a problem.

psychological commentary prepared by staff psychologist

Intellectually, Cora functions in the average range, though this appears reduced from her optimal intellectual capacity as a function of a significant depressive quality and a concommitant reduction in response time. There is a certain impulsivity (sic) that is used in an effort to avoid the ruminative aspects and the unproductive features associated with the depression.

Prior to the speech therapy, we note an intense agitation in handling the projective materials. There is a dysphoric quality, a tendency to be somewhat labile emotionally, and an immature tendency that fails to come to terms with mature needs and impulses. She is afraid of interpersonal relationships and tends to be isolated and introversive.

Immediately following the speech therapy, we find a marked diminution in the hysterical and hypochondriacal qualities present in this woman and a reduction in the depression from a highly significant level to, at most, one of moderate extent. She is considerably less socially isolated and considerably more able to deal with the aggressive motives that are characteristic of adult interactions.

After the speech program, Cora seemed somewhat more introversive, but considerably less overwhelmed by the necessity to maintain obsessive and compulsive defenses which should make her day-to-day functioning meaningfully more efficient.

concluding comments

I think the therapeutic relationship was important in this

client's success. Cora was able to identify with the clinician who was a female of about the same age. Both of them were rather tall women. Cora enjoyed being with the clinician. Subsequently, as therapy proceeded, the client adopted the clinician's calm attitude of considering several possible ways of interpreting experiences and memories. I think the matching of client and clinician was very important in Cora's progress. In addition, as she found it possible to discuss her opinions and feelings with her clinicians and the members of the group (her speech was improving as she learned modifications) this more open and comfortable attitude generalized to situations outside the clinic. As mentioned in the previous discussion, Cora was able to discover some of the things people thought about her at the present rather than generalizing from earlier experiences. Of course, it cannot be overlooked that the process occurring was an interaction between the clearing up of mis-evaluations and the possibility that the people in Cora's environment were reacting to her differently as change in her social attitudes and speech behavior occurred.

The reinforcement from the group was also important to Cora, and it seemed to us that her progress might not have been as great in another group in which there may have been a different reaction to her as a person. As research in psychotherapy has indicated, the effects of reinforcement are closely related to the relationship in therapy. I think that Cora's progress in all of the different areas of therapy including change of attitude and reduction of fear and avoidance behavior was greatly influenced by the relationship she had with the individual clinician, the group clinician, and her fellow clients.

Cora brought to therapy an analytic, rational attitude toward problems related to her work, and we were able to manage therapy so that she applied this problem solving attitude to herself.

A CLINICAL FAILURE: FRED
CLINICIAN: HUGO GREGORY

Fred was an 18-year-old, white male, short and muscular in physique, who was a freshman in college. The first impression was that he looked insecure and childish and walked and moved in a way that was immature. He sat in a stiff, tense posture, with the head usually tilted to one side. He lived at home with his mother and father. Fred stated that his father was unable to work due to poor physical health.

The client was a severe stutterer (oftentimes he blocked on every other word in conversational speech). He stuttered mostly on initial sounds, but there was also blocking on medial and final syllables of words. He displayed considerable tension of the lips, tongue, jaw, and larynx as he spoke. Starters such as "uh," "wa wa wa," and "well uh" were used frequently. A gasping type inhalation was involved in approximately one of every three blocks. Breaking through a speech block was sometimes accompanied by a slight leg movement. Fluent words, or occasional fluent phrases, were spoken in a slow, labored rate. The lack of motor facility of the speech mechanism was apparent even before an oral examination was done. The same general quality of incoordination appeared to characterize all of Fred's body movements (hand movements, walking, etc.).

Diadochokinetic rates of the tongue were slow. There was improvement of diadochokinetic rates as the examination progressed from tongue tip, to lingua velar, to laryngeal level. "Kah Luh" was easier for him to do than was "Tuh Kah." Tongue tip movements improved when the jaw was stabilized. There was considerable deterioration in the precision of articulation when the rate of producing "Puh Tuh Kuh" was increased. Reversals of "Kuh" and "Tuh" occured on "Puh Tuh Kuh." There was a slight extensor thrust movement of the tongue when the rate of tongue lateralization was increased. One point and two point sensory discrimination of the face and tongue appeared normal.

Fred said that he had stuttered as long as he could remember. Fred's mother recalled that the subject's speech development was slow—first words at about two years—still not using good sentences when he went to kindergarten. (According to the mother, the subject walked alone at 11 months.) The interview with the mother also revealed that the client had speech therapy in the first grade and then "off and on when it was available." The mother reported that she had been a stutterer but that she had stopped stuttering when

18 years of age. However, observation of the mother revealed mild to moderate stuttering characterized mainly by rapid repetitions and prolongations of vowels.

Fred was seen two hours a week in individual therapy and two hours a week in group sessions for nine months. Therapy began with a case history. During these discussion oriented interviews, the clinician's objective was to establish an atmosphere in which the client would feel that we were interested in him as a person and wanted to understand his problem. Such questions were discussed as the following: What do you think caused your problem? What have you been told will help stutterers? What have you done for your stuttering?

These same topics were discussed in the group sessions. Fred brought out the possibility of heredity as a cause because he said his mother had told him she stuttered until she was 18. Although Fred was the youngest client in the group of ten, he contributed freely. On several occasions he brought up topics which led to fruitful discussions. For example, he stated that all non-fluency was stuttering. This resulted in a discussion of people's fluency in general and whether or not others who were disfluent had the same feeling, *i.e.* fear, related to it, as does a stutterer. Some ideas offered by Fred were: "A person may lose eye contact because he is embarrassed." When talking about relaxation, he said to the group, "I think you have to think relaxed." When talking about speech fluency, he said, "Maybe every child is at one time non-fluent, and if a child notices this non-fluency the child begins to avoid it." These points are mentioned because in the staffings there was discussion among the clinicians about the value of the content of the client's statements and attitude when talking in the group. He seemed to be enjoying the group a great deal. He would "grab" an opportunity to correct one of the other client's statements. The individual clinician was of the opinion that these statements, such as the above quotes, represented a repeating of what others said. The clinician was concerned that Fred showed very little ability to integrate ideas and to reason. It was apparent that to some extent the other clients were amused and, perhaps, annoyed at times with the "childish glee" which seemed present when these comments were made.

The decision was made in staffing that the clinician would discuss the purpose of the group and the importance of thinking about a contribution before hand—is it adding to the discussion, is it monopolizing the discussion? After this, it was observed that the client began to daydream in the group just as he had been observed to do in individual sessions. Evidently, we increased anxiety and brought about this behavior which was his way of coping with frustration and conflict. Consequently, we questioned our approach. We speculated that it would have been wiser to let the group reaction develop, as we have done on other occasions, and then in individual therapy help him explore the reasons for the group reaction and his feelings about it. I think the immaturity aspect, as contrasted with the more frequently encountered hostile or "know it all" attitude, was what misled us. I think we had a need to tell "the little boy" too soon. Possibly this was a demonstration of our attitude toward "childish problems." We had recognized that one of our principal goals with Fred was to help him develop the use of his higher mental processes, but we did not adopt a strategy that would shape the kind of thinking of which he was then capable (as represented by his verbalizations) into the kind of thinking we perceived he needed to do.

The first meeting of the group at which the clients were asked to bring a relative or friend was held toward the close of two months of therapy. The client was encouraged to bring his mother in keeping with the belief that those in the client's environment needed to know what was transpiring in therapy and, furthermore, that they needed to know what changes in behavior to reinforce. The client's mother was verbose and domineering. Although it was not expected that the clients would have shared much of what was ocurring at the clinic with those at home at this early stage of therapy, it was apparent after this meeting that Fred had not told his mother anything about the group and that, furthermore, he never did talk with her about himself unless she urged him to do so. The mother attempted, within the range of the subject's hearing, to tell us about her son's "emotional problems." She related that he laughed when he shouldn't, that he jumped up and got excited while watching TV, paced the floor, etc. At the next individual session, the client said, "My mother talked to you about what she called emotional problems, and I would like to talk about these things for a few minutes." He said that his daydreaming bothered his mother and then said, "I can't figure out if this is right or wrong." He went on to point out that "what bothers her is she talks to me, and I may not hear her." He told how he liked to fantasy that he was a coach and that in his room at home he would talk out loud to the team. (Fred's one success in life appeared to be his cross country running, and he wanted to major in physical education and be an athletic coach). He said he enjoyed this fantasy and thought it all right in his room.

Two months later after another visit by the mother to the clinic the client said of his parents, "They don't care how my speech gets better. They just want it to get better." Later, he said, "There is a personality conflict between my parents. You see they don't like each other. First time my father threw something was when I was seven years old. Last August was the last time, and since a son shouldn't beat up his father . . ." In addition, the mother refers to the fellows who participate in cross country running as "animals." He described this home situation as causing his tension.

We saw clearly now that we could not expect support from the client's home. In fact, the wisdom of trying to explain any of the therapy procedure to the mother was questioned. These visits to the group by the mother helped us to understand the client's previous learning environment and present situation, but we speculated that it might have been better to interview the mother privately and make some determination of our therapeutic strategy as to whether or not to involve her in therapy process. The question arises as to whether it is advisable for a parent like this to be involved at all, thinking she is informed when she is not able to cooperate constructively. This client's situation made us reconsider carefully this aspect of our approach to therapy.

Meanwhile, therapeutic activities aimed at analyzing and modifying Fred's avoidance behaviors (secondary symptoms) were underway. The clinician hoped to relate self-awareness of speech to awareness of self in general. Negative practice (imitating actual stuttering pattern) was used in the individual sessions. Fred began to realize what he was doing when the speech flow was interrupted. The mirror and tape recorder were used as Fred learned to watch his stuttering pattern and listen to those auditory aspects such as starters. Negative practice began with work on the starters, head jerks, and the gasping patterns of breathing. He was very pleased to be able to demonstrate some of the negative practice in the group. Relaxation procedures were taught.

Fred was very cooperative in carrying out the suggested modification procedures, such as the slide, bounce, and delayed response. Progress as compared to the others in the group was considered satisfactory. However, he demonstrated very little ability to evaluate a speech response or procedure and to generalize from one *specific* act of speech modification to another. He had difficulty using a variety of modifications and, thus, getting a feeling of being able to do first one thing and then another with his speech. We worked on improving the motor activity of the tongue and integrated this with the work on making a smooth transition in voluntary stuttering.

The client's speech at the clinic was improved considerably after six months of therapy, and he reported successes in using modification outside the clinic. A regression was observed after his mother's second visit to the clinic. Fred also reported that he was feeling apathetic. He attributed this feeling to not having competed in a race for four months (as mentioned previously this appeared to be his only real accomplishment) and having stuttered "just as bad as before in talking to a teacher."

In the continuing discussion of his attitudes and feelings the daydreaming was interpreted as being, in part, that type of activity in which all people indulge, and, in part, a way of coping with the frustration he felt about his speech and the situation at home. Other "adjustment mechanisms" such as rationalization and compensation were discussed in the group and individual sessions, but the use of these labels in his thinking came very slowly.

As the nine month therapy program came to a close, Fred was feeling rather good about his new speech pattern. He was using pull-outs and preparatory sets. He thought that work on phrasing had been particularly helpful. During the mother's last visit to the clinic, the clinician attempted to commend Fred's good work in studying and modifying his speech. The mother winked at the clinician and said, "You deserve all the credit."

The client's mother called me four months after the end of therapy, when Fred was due home from college for a visit, to say he would like a conference with me. The mother said, "He is stuttering terribly." Fred called my home when I was away and when I returned, my daughter said, "Some little boy who stutters very badly called you." I saw Fred and heard his report that he was having considerable trouble in all situations. Even though he stuttered rather severely, the gasping inhalation which was a part of the pattern before therapy was not observed. Fred said he was thinking that he should not stay away at school. One reason given for this was that his cross country running was not as good, and he thought he might lose his scholarship, but in addition, he thought his mother would rather have him at home.

psychological commentary by staff psychologist

Though Fred has completed at least two years of a college program, we note that on the Wechsler Adult Intelligence Scale he obtains a Full-Scale IQ score of only 97. He is functioning on the tests at a level well below what might be considered his optimal intellectual capacity, for we find a highly significant variability on the individual subtests in which he misses quite easy items while answering correctly much more difficult material with relative ease. He is highly pedantic and quite rigid in his use of the intellectual ability, showing no flexibility or ease in calling forth the potential. He deals with the tasks as if quite unable to evaluate the adequacy of his own functioning as a result of the constricting and impoverishing defenses.

On the projective tests administered immediately prior to the speech therapy program, Fred shows profound feelings of inadequacy, inferiority and worthlessness. In completing the heading on the test form, he writes "boy" in the space for *sex*. There is a profoundly depressive quality that is avoided full conscious recognition by the investment of quite massive amounts of energy in terms of repressive defenses. It is this quality that we see revealed on the intellectual material as resulting in a notable impotence and impoverishment in the utilization of the intellectual potential. In relationships with people, Fred, during the pre-therapy period, seems obsequious, self-demeaning, and self-derogating. There is a significant passive-dependent quality in the character structure.

Upon the completion of the speech therapy program, we find meaningful psychological change s, some enhancing the negative self-concept, some showing an attempt to make changes in overt behavior, as if attempting to change what he realizes is inappropriate and self-defeating behavior. For example, the negative traits regarding feelings of worthlessness and inadequacy are significantly enhanced after the therapy program, as if Fred has become aware of the full impact of these attributes in the psychological organization. Concomitantly, we see increments in his desires to achieve and in a certain aggressiveness in day-to-day activities. These positive qualities account for the reduction in the marked depression that was present pre-therapy, but considerably less so after the speech program; the aggressive and hard-driving qualities also account for the reduction in the fear of interpersonal relationships.

concluding comments

There were many significant factors operating in Fred's stuttering problem:

We were able to identify organic components of the problem portrayed in his generally poor motor coordination and the specific deficits in the motor control of the tongue, lips, and laryngeal valving mechanism. The psychosocial factors were of such great magnitude to require a long term program of psychotherapy. We became increasingly aware of this as therapy continued. We will continue to follow Fred, and, hopefully, additional speech therapy, combined with a psychotherapy program, can be arranged. At present, he is attending college in another state.

I think the client's therapeutic experience could have been better if we had been more accepting of his contributions to the group early in therapy—attaching more importance to the positive experience it was for him to be able to talk in a group and say what he pleased. We talk about the importance of this in counterconditioning and anxiety reduction, but we did not react as appropriately as we should in this situation. It is my impression that his intelligence (WAIS I.Q. 97) combined with his environmental experiences which have not encouraged maturity limited his ability to evaluate himself and his social behavior.

We have questioned the advisability of placing Fred in this group. It may be that a pattern of therapy in which at first he would have received individual therapy only, followed by group therapy after it was seen that he could profit from and contribute to the group process would have been a more successful approach.

I think we should have evaluated the parental environmental influences differently. We assessed the home environments at the time we brought the mother into the group situation to give her information about the therapeutic process. In some adult situations, of which the present client's may be illustrative, we may want to control carefully the information the parents or wife have about therapy. Fred's main work in therapy may have to be to learn to react differently to the environment rather than hoping that along with his change there will be change in environmental factors.

Finally, the psychological commentary indicates that some constructive personality changes did occur. At my last conference with Fred (three months after therapy ended) he was able, during a one hour interview, to begin modifying his speech behavior fairly well, once again, although he stuttered severely at the beginning of the hour. Consequently, the prognosis now, as compared to before therapy, is somewhat better.

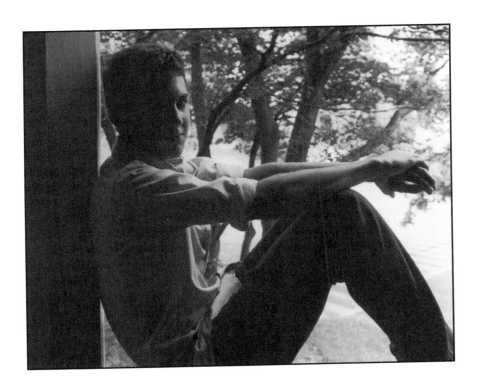

A CLINICAL SUCCESS: STEVE
CLINICIAN: HAROLD L. LUPER

Steve is a 30-year-old college student who came to see me about his stuttering this year. He is married and a father. His marriage appears to be successful though there are minor conflicts between him and his wife and some difficulty in role adjustment in marriage. Steve is almost over-conscientious in most activities—apparently due to the fact that he has high goals but feels he is not superior. Steve's stuttering on the first examination was quite mild in severity but frequent in occurrence. Almost all of his disfluencies were double repetitions of initial sounds accompanied by a mild degree of tension in the articulators. He used few if any avoidances or tricks. He spoke freely and had a pleasant manner.

During the first interview, Steve described his speech problem as quite severe (and he frequently repeated this evaluation). He felt that his stuttering interfered greatly with his present schooling and with his future vocational plans. He stated that he had stuttered since childhood. For a time, he said he had stuttered in a more severe fashion, but on his own he learned to repress the severe occurrences by retrials on difficult sounds. He was maintaining satisfactory academic grades (high C's) but wanted to do much better. He worked long hours at a campus cafeteria. He had withdrawn from college in his sophomore year for financial reasons, returning after spending several years in the Army. He was active in church and played the accordian semi-professionally.

After one or two exploratory sessions, therapy was structured to emphasize a working relationship directed toward helping him understand why he tensed up as he talked. Since his stuttering behavior appeared so mild, little stress was given to teaching "controls." For motivational purposes, the carrot of "learning to control your tensions so you will have less difficulty" was dangled before him. Perhaps it would be closer to the truth to say that Steve expressed a strong desire for the quick cure, but I felt this approach was more appropriate than one providing a technique for eliminating the stuttering.

Steve was quite a talker and was easily self-hypnotized into statements about all the good he was getting from therapy. His loquaciousness sometimes made it difficult to keep the topic of conversation within those areas that seemed most productive. In general, however, he cooperated fully in these exploratory sessions and at no time did his talkativeness appear to be a way to avoid vital issues.

Early in therapy he was given Wendell Johnson's "Stuttering and What You Can Do About It" for reading. This formed a basis for several discussions. Steve read the book, was quite impressed by this approach, and apparently understood it correctly. Discussions centered around the content of the book with frequent applications to his own situation. I questioned him about vital concepts, listened, and reinforced "correct" interpretations and applications. Several sessions were devoted to his seeking to incorporate some of the ideas into his speech behavior. As the frequency of his stuttering remained about the same, it was decided that a direct attempt to modify the repetitions was in order. I urged him to go directly into difficult words and prolong the sound with reduced tension. Experience with this practice brought out the fact that he frequently was unaware of his stuttering until after it occurred and that his overall "bodily tonicity" appeared to be the predominant factor in changes in fluency level. Consequently, we spent several sessions analyzing how he felt (how tense, how relaxed, etc.) as he talked and then instituted a procedure of his learning to "fake" different tonicity states and to shift from a tense to a relaxed tension state (overall bodily tension). Eventually, we found that when he deliberately slowed down his speaking rate and consciously adopted a more relaxed bodily tension level, his disfluencies reduced to near zero. In essence we were using an old device we warn patients against—that is, stopping or slowing down to prevent stuttering. This worked remarkedly well!

After several successful situations in modifying his stuttering frequency level—both in and out of the clinic—we found that his stuttering would increase again unless he was continually thinking about working on it. We decided, therefore, to return to a study of factors that increased his overall tension and that made him more likely to be tense. Therapy now entered more of a psychotherapy counseling situation. Whereas during the previous stages, I had suggested techniques or reinforced appropriate solutions he suggested, I now encouraged him to talk about possible sources of tension. I listened and praised his insights and tentative hypotheses. Therapy continued for several weeks in which he discovered that he tended to have unrealistic aspirations for himself, he felt that others were expecting a great deal from him, and he ventilated some negative feelings toward family, self, and wife. At times, we would again work on controlling bodily tension, but most sessions were spent in talking out problems, re-examining them objectively, and making insights or tentative hypotheses about their effect on his total tension level and his speech.

Overall, my role with Steve was essentially didactic and supportive. I was more didactic when working directly on speech. I served as an interpreter and clarifier during most of the discussions concerning problems of adjustment. After two quarters of therapy, he and I agreed that further direct therapy was not needed at this time, since he was generally experiencing success in speaking, was gaining an understanding of what made him tense and what he could do about it, and was altering some of his basic attitudes of over-expectation in terms of personal performance. He was asked to return from time to time to let me know how he was doing. The last time I saw him was when he dropped by six months following therapy to let me know he was still doing well.

Why was Steve successful in therapy? As I look back over Steve's therapy, I believe there are several reasons. In the first place, his problem was not as severe as many others with whom I've worked. But I believe there were other factors more important. Steve worked hard at all he did. He was mature, and he came to therapy with a willingness to do his part. Furthermore, he was coping successfully with most areas of his life. It was a financial hardship to stay in school, but he was doing it and without having given up outside activities.

Would any therapy approach have worked just as well? I doubt it. I believe he was a person "made for" Johnson's semantogenic approach (as contrasted to Elaine, my failure case, who liked to think this explained her stuttering). His unrealistically high expectation levels created tensions and anxieties. He made a mountain of anxiety out of a molehill of speech disfluencies. As he read Johnson's book, he came to see that he did not have to be perfect and that there were other ways to look at himself and his problems. The semantogenic approach helped him to convert his amorphous anxiety-producing concerns into solvable problems.

I also believe that the direct work on speech which we entered into later in therapy was necessary. In a sense, he had to put some of his new attitudes to test. The rapid success with simple modification techniques reinforced this new view about stuttering and problem solving. Since the stuttering symptoms were simple, the needed modification techniques were also simple. I don't think that telling himself to slow down and take it easy would have worked if he had had many severe secondary symptoms.

Some of our most productive sessions occurred after he had found that his stuttering increased again unless he was constantly thinking about it. I believe this experience helped him to see that speaking fluently was not just a mechanical matter—although he had learned that he, himself, had the ability to speak in a fluent manner. The attitudes he had previously accepted from the semantogenic approach and the success he had made in speaking fluently when being careful supported him now as he examined more closely those factors in his life that made him tense up and that robbed him of his confidence.

There are probably many other reasons why Steve's therapy

was successful, but I feel that the two major reasons were his own readiness for therapy and his compatibility with the therapy program offered.

A CLINICAL FAILURE: ELAINE
CLINICIAN: HAROLD L. LUPER

A few years ago I was contacted by a public school therapis in our city about a teacher who had a severe stuttering problem. The therapist indicated that this person was quite withdrawn and very sensitive about her difficulty. The therapist had talked to her several times about entering therapy and had finally persuaded her to come for an interview with me to discuss the possibilities.

A few days later, Elaine appeared for her first interview. She was a very masculine female—30 years of age. When she stuttered—which was quite often—she would drop her head, look embarrassed and wait for help. She indicated she had had no previous therapy—either speech or psychotherapy, although she had read several books about stuttering. She indicated that from these readings she had decided that her problem was best explained by Johnson's semantogenic theory.

During this interview, Elaine indicated that she had stuttered since childhood but felt that the problem was worse now than at anytime previously. She taught young children primarily because she felt they were more accepting than were high school students about her speech difficulties.

Elaine expressed strong concerns about entering therapy, indicating that she would be embarrassed for anyone to know that she was receiving therapy and that she hated to put herself in the position of one who had to be helped. She was, however, concerned by her speech problem and felt something needed to be done. We set up an appointment for two weeks later, and I asked her to let me know by that time whether or not she would enter therapy. When she returned two weeks later, she stated that she did wish to try it, although she had reservations.

Several sessions were spent in exploring her background, her stuttering, her present attitudes, and in my seeking to convince her of the importance of facing instead of running away from the problem of stuttering. During these discussions, it became apparent that she was inclined to take a detached intellectual approach to self-analysis and to quote frequently from well-known writers in speech pathology and psychology.

Individual weekly sessions were held with Elaine for the next two months during which time she appeared to be making a little progress in terms of accepting her speech difficulty, although she still exhibited an abnormally high degree of resistance to change and sensitivity about her problem. I began to feel that she could make changes in her speech but that she needed another therapist. I couldn't break through the resistance and the intellectual veneer.

I decided to shift therapy to a female graduate student who was the "mother type." My thinking was that Elaine was a person who had been severely restricted in her contacts with others and who needed to build up a basically healthy relationship with someone. Since she appeared to be resistant toward doing this with a male therapist, a warm female therapist was thought more appropriate. The therapist was instructed to be permissive, accepting, and to try to increase Elaine's spontaneity in expressing herself as much as possible. She was also instructed to see if she couldn't get Elaine moving in terms of making changes in her speech. I felt she needed some "positive speaking experiences."

Therapy sessions continued with this female therapist for six months. During this time, Elaine made some progress, but never a great deal. She reported that she was gradually entering into feared situations and was having some success in conquering some of them. She also became a little more spontaneous in speaking with the therapist and with other persons around the Center.

Two problems began showing up at this time:

1. More and more, Elaine demanded that she, rather than the therapist, determine the course of therapy for each session. I realize that Carl Rogers would approve of such an approach (in fact, she repeatedly quoted him); however, this began to develop into a period where we felt no change was being made. It was almost as if Elaine were taking advantage of the time of the therapist to satisfy her own needs for female companionship and a good listener. Whenever we began to suggest directions to the conversation, she claimed we were not allowing self-determination of goals.

2. Elaine also began displaying strong inappropriate, hostile reactions to other staff members around the clinic. She would complain that some did things which were damaging to her self-image as a person with a speech problem. Most of the instances had little basis in fact, and, from what we could make out, they seldom appeared to be true representations of the intentions of the "doer of the unjust act."

In addition, some of the ways that the therapist finally found to work with Elaine seemed rather unusual. For example, Elaine constantly demanded stars as rewards for doing a good job in modifying her speech. This kind of reward for an educated adult definitely seemed unusual. (Later when Elaine was transferred to another therapist, she complained about the new therapist and commented that "she will not give me any stars for words that I handle well.") Throughout most of the time that the student therapist was working with her, Elaine tended to direct the therapy sessions, to give herself speech assignments and to show a small degree of improvement in terms of modifying her speech pattern. But no real strong gains were seen and, at the end of the summer quarter when the therapist was ready to graduate, Elaine seemed quite threatened by the fact that her therapist was leaving. She also felt dissatisfied with her progress and decided she would discontinue therapy. It took strong urging from myself and from the student therapist to get her to remain in therapy and to transfer to a new therapist. We finally convinced her to continue coming for awhile and give it a trial. I found myself urging more strongly than I normally would, since I felt the progress that she had begun to make might not be continued once she left therapy and since I felt that more progress could probably be made at this time with a different therapist. It seemed to me then that the warm motherly type had outlived her usefulness anyway since she was unable to help Elaine move beyond the point of dependence and self-indulgence.

I should mention here that I never got the feeling that Elaine was making a real effort in therapy. She would take on a task, such as learning to modify her stuttering by use of "pullouts", but was seldom willing to stick with it long enough to gain any competency. She would very quickly fail and then spend the rest of the session explaining why she was unable to make progress. I always had the feeling that her efforts were half-hearted, that either she had such a tremendous amount of tension that she felt completely helpless or that she did not really want to make progress. I also had some doubts about the therapist I had assigned to work with her. This was her first stuttering case, and even though she was an intelligent girl and appeared to have quite a good understanding of how to work with stutterers, I kept having the feeling that she was simply being too weak herself, and this was really what led to Elaine's control of the therapy situation.

So therapy continued with a new therapist—again a female, but one who was not so permissive nor accepting as the therapist who had been working with her for several months. The new therapist did not share my philosophies about working with stutterers. She tended to look upon all problems as deep psychosexual conflicts and wanted to force the therapy as quickly as possible into this kind of structure. My own feeling at this time was that, although I realized that Elaine had what I considered pretty deep hurts because of her years of severe speech problems, she was not ready for deep psychosexual counseling. I felt that we needed to help Elaine make more improvement in the solution of her speech problem before attempting to get into deeper therapy and that if deeper therapy were needed, it would best be done by a qualified psychologist or psychiatrist.

The new therapist, however, did push the issue and after one or two sessions, Elaine asked for an appointment with me where she stated she felt threatened by the new approach, and she wanted to know whether or not I felt psychological counseling was needed. My answer to her was that I felt that psychological problems quite frequently were associated with stuttering, but that I felt she needed to work directly on her speech at this time. As she left the room, I knew I had made a mistake.

During this same time we began an evening adult stuttering group. I am afraid the group was badly mismatched and simply never jelled. Elaine came once or twice but then refused to come further. She began, at this time, to attempt to play one therapist against another. She became friends with several of the therapists in the Center and would go to them and ask them for the solution to her problem. She would tend to put each one in the role of disapproving of the others' suggestion for therapy. She also expressed great hostility toward some of the therapists in the group, once or twice concerning events which I had witnessed and which I felt were very inappropriately judged by her. With the great increase in hostility which began showing up at this time, and, perhaps, reacting somewhat to the pressure of the new female therapist who wanted to administer deep psychosexual counseling, I decided that I did need to have a good psychological evaluation before continuing further. I, therefore, called Elaine in and indicated that we could not continue speech therapy until we had a psychological evaluation and clearance. Elaine refused, but continued to try to play one member of the staff against the other. She would call members at home and write letters to her former therapist indicating that we had taken away her therapy and were unwilling to help her any more. I insisted that my last decision be maintained; that is, that she not be continued in therapy until we had received psychological clearance and further psychological information. I offered to help her make an appointment for such an evaluation, but she refused to do anything more about it.

Why was I unable to help Elaine? Partially because she prevented it. Perhaps therapy would have been unsuccessful even if I had made no mistakes. But I made plenty. For example, this was probably a case that I should not have assigned to a student. I should have foreseen that she would be threatened when the therapist finished school. I could tell this was a problem needing a deep satisfying relationship with a therapist, and yet I assigned her to someone who would soon not be available.

I'm afraid I missed a real opportunity the day she came to me complaining about the psychosexual approach and asking if psychotherapy were needed. That was the turning point. I should have utilized this opportunity to refer her then—not later after I became frustrated. I'm afraid I let a theoretical argument over how best to work with stutterers interfere with my judgment. I became defensive and thus created a situation from which I could not later withdraw without creating antagonism and lack of confidence in my therapeutic ability.

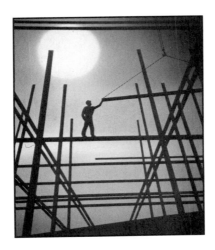

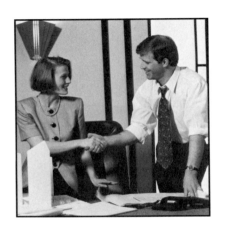

A CLINICAL SUCCESS: LOUISE
CLINICIAN: FRANK B. ROBINSON

Louise, an attractive and stylishly dressed 35-year-old divorcee, came to the clinic at the suggestion of a Vocational Rehabilitation counsellor who earlier had arranged for her to attend a school to prepare her to be a dental assistant. Since the completion of the training, she had been working for a year. She was unhappy with her job because of the working conditions, but she felt that her speech would prevent her from keeping any other employment. She had had no previous treatment for her stuttering. She said she had always been told by her mother that it was something she could stop if she wanted to and that her husband to whom she was married for thirteen years had told her the same thing. She also said that a psychiatrist to whom she had gone for help with problems associated with the final breakup of her marriage had told her that the stuttering was just a symptom of unresolved emotional problems, and it would not be profitable to work on it directly.

The stuttering was severe and frequent. It was characterized by prolonged struggle behavior, tremors, and numerous repeated attempts to initiate the beginning sounds or syllables of troublesome words. Word and situation avoidance occurred only infrequently. Louise reported going through several phases in which she worked to hide the stuttering with substitutions and careful phrasing and by avoiding feared situations when she could, but she said it never really worked out well. She said she got tired of trying to think up ways of talking to avoid stuttering and there were too many situations to avoid. She didn't want to become a recluse. In fact, she said that she really liked to talk, so she had become reconciled to the stuttering and just tried to avoid thinking about "the awful faces" she made when it occurred.

Louise said that she had some recollection of stuttering occasionally in the early grades in school but that it was no problem until the junior high years. It apparently had become much worse then. She would not recite in classes and her grades, which up to that time had been a source of great pride for her, became the cause of much frustration and embarrassment. This pattern continued through high school. She even failed one course because she refused to present an oral report.

highlights of life history

Louise's parents were divorced when she was six. There were

two other children, boys, both younger than Louise. All remained with the mother who arranged to live with a widowed and childless brother who provided a home for them, but, according to Louise, did not like children.

The mother remarried when Louise was eight years old. She said that the step-father was essentially a kind man who tried to be good to the children, but that she was always afraid of him. She later concluded that it was because her mother was always reminding the children about being quiet. She suspected her mother did this out of fear of losing the security her husband provided, but Louise somehow got the idea that it was because her step-father did not like noisy children.

It was during that same year that Louise was accidentally hit in the face with a baseball bat and damaged some permanent front teeth. She had to have some rather extensive surgery and for some time afterwards she said she could remember her mother introducing her as "and this is our ugly duckling." As a consequence of her experiences that particular year, Louise recalled being utterly miserable. She didn't like school, she hated her brothers for teasing her about her teeth, and she was afraid of her step-father.

Despite her problems, Louise did very well in school. She had perfect records on three occasions, and she remembered being very happy about the academic successes. As she told it, "I was really proud of that. It was the one place I could excell, and it really hurt me when I got to junior high school and didn't get good grades anymore. It was just too embarrassing to talk. I always scored high on I.Q. tests, though, and, for some reason, I was always popular with the boys, too. I never really understood that. I kept my teeth hidden behind a sober face, but I still felt ugly and the way the stuttering contorted my face made it worse. And then I developed a sarcastic attitude. I had a very sharp tongue and enjoyed using it to cut people down to size. But I still always got along all right with the boys."

When Louise was a junior, her grandfather on her father's side died and left each of the three children some money. Much to her surprise, Louise told us, her mother allowed the children to have the money. Louise used some of hers to buy some nice clothes, and she said that she has always dressed well since. She said, "I have never felt pretty, but I have always looked good."

After high school, Louise worked for a year and a half as a gift wrapper in a department store. She then married a man she met on a blind date. She said she was overwhelmed by his worldly manner. He was a gambler and quite a heavy drinker. But he always had money, and Louise was impressed with the way he made it and the way he spent it. They lived on a farm owned by his parents. They paid no rent and his parents also paid all the fuel and utility bills.

In spite of what seemed like an ideal arrangement, the marriage was a bust almost from the beginning. Her husband was an only child, and Louise said that he was really tied to his parents, who, in time, were running the lives of "their children." There was a child, a boy. Louise told us, "I adored that boy, and I would have left sooner if I had felt that I could support the two of us. I finally did get a job in a war production plant and wanted to leave then. But he wouldn't let me, and his parents thought it would be a terrible way for me to treat him and them after all they had done for me."

Then Louise became involved with another married man. Things got worse fast. Her husband still would not let her leave him, she lost her job when the plant suddenly shut down, she feared she could not get another job because of the stuttering. Her mother was claiming that she was not being a proper wife and mother, and his parents were no longer speaking to her. She discussed the matter with her physician who arranged for her to talk with a psychiatrist who, in turn, arranged for some vocational guidance.

After she began working, Louise said that conditions at home continued to worsen. She finally left and got a divorce and custody of the child.

When she came to the clinic, she was still going with the married man. She claimed they were very much in love and that she felt really loved for the first time in her life. However, he didn't want to leave his family unless he could have his two children, and his wife had said she would never agree to that.

appraisal and treatment approach

As someone who became an example of successful therapy, we have had few cases who appeared to be less likely candidates. We have seldom encountered a case who was involved in a more tangled web of marital and other personal conflicts or who had an early history that more clearly suggested an association between stuttering and psychological problems. Louise had marked feelings of insecurity, of inadequacy, and of guilt about the mess she had made of her life. The prognosis appeared only fair at best. We felt that any treatment directed to the stuttering behavior would have little chance of satisfactory stability without supplementary psychotherapy, and that that might well involve fairly long term treatment by a psychiatrist. We certainly would not have predicted that four years after a treatment experience that focussed on the conscious acquisition of a controlled form of stuttering, this woman would report to us that she was happily married, maintaining a job as a receptionist in a large firm of corporation lawyers, and that her stuttering, although occasionally troublesome for telephone calls and an intercom system, was generally considered no problem.

The treatment involved participation in three group meetings each week with four other adult stutterers, all men, a weekly individual meeting with the therapist, and assigned projects which usually were done in company with one of the other stutterers. The group meetings were used to present information about stuttering, to clarify the goals and specific treatment techniques, to report and share experiences, and for experimenting with techniques related to the treatment. The major emphasis of the treatment was on the acquisition of a controlled form of stuttering. The fact that Louise was the only female in the group was not a specifically planned arrangement. The four men were the others who had applied and been accepted for treatment of that time. We considered the wisdom of having one female in such a group. Sometimes such an arrangement can have a distinctly adverse effect on treatment. In this instance, however, we did not think this would be true, particularly because Louise had a history of "getting along all right with the boys." She was also older and in many ways more mature than the others in the group. Also, there were two others in the group who were in their twenties and who, like her, had not gone to college.

results and follow-up

Louise proved to be a good participant. She was verbal, witty, and insightful. She reveled in the all-male company and enjoyed the experience of "being in college." However, although she participated willingly in projects to explore her own stuttering behavior and her attitudes about it, the involvement for the first several weeks was superficial. She preferred talking about it. Then, almost overnight, she began to participate actively. She became willing to test the validity of her feelings about being a stutterer and to confront and explore ways of modifying the stuttering behavior. She even agreed to initiate a discussion in the group about her teeth, and did so, and discovered none of the other people had noticed anything unusual.

We, of course, were very pleased with the change. We assumed it was a reflection of a common occurrence in therapy. There is almost always some resistance to a direct confrontation with the stuttering behavior and to the therapy process in general until the stutterer can have some feeling of assurance that what he is being advised to do not only makes sense but will also actually help him. This is what we supposed had happened in this case. Some weeks later, because we had some curiosity about the unusual abruptness of the change, we asked Louise about that happening. She was very definite in her answer. She said it had been due to the profound effects of a book I had suggested to the group one day as a good one to read about stuttering. It was Wendell Johnson's *People in Quandaries*. She said, "That book hit me right between the eyes," and that everything we had been discussing suddenly became clear to her.

Louise began to have some success in controlling the stuttering behavior, and the discovery that she could voluntarily control the stuttering and thereby eliminate the hated cosmetic effect provided patent reinforcement for further effort. She progressed rapidly. She became the bell cow of the group. Additional reinforcement came from comments from her friends, her employer, and her boy-friend. She bloomed. And she became almost free from any noticeable stuttering except for telephone situations and at times at the beginnings of conversations.

One day the role of guilt in stuttering was discussed in the group, and in some subsequent individual sessions, Louise initiated further discussion on the subject. The stuttering was notably more difficult to control in these sessions, but later she claimed that they were the most valuable sessions we had.

Her freedom from troublesome stuttering continued through the remainder of the clinic program. During the last few weeks she talked about seeking a different job. She also mentioned leaving town. She expressed hopelessness about the situation with her boy-friend and thought it would be best to make a clean break to a new environment. She had relatives in a distant community and took several days for a visit. When she returned she reported that her stuttering remained under satisfactory control and that she was going to go there to stay.

She did leave and for awhile sent weekly reports. She got a job in a medical clinic and got along all right for four months. Then a public address system was installed and "all hell broke loose."

The severe stuttering returned in full force and no reports came for several weeks. Then she wrote to say that she was all right again, though on occasion she still "stuttered miserably on that damn intercom." She said she had contemplated coming to see us and then decided that she would first try and regain control of her stuttering herself. "I just made myself work on it. I decided I had too much to lose now. I didn't want to have to return a failure." Later that first year she had two other experiences with sieges of troublesome stuttering. One occurred when her ex-boyfriend came to town suddenly and said he couldn't get along without her and was going to leave his wife and come down with her. The second one took place when her former husband came to try and talk her into coming back with him.

Also during the latter part of that first year she wrote to tell about her new boyfriend, a thirty-year-old bachelor professor of philosophy in a local university. Later they were married and reports came less frequently. The general tenor was of satisfaction with life and with her ability to manage the stuttering when she felt it was sufficiently important to do so. And on other occasions, although the stuttering continued to annoy her, it was no longer a source of worry, embarrassment, or guilt.

We believe this example of a clinical success illustrates several important things about therapy with stutterers. First, it illustrates how a problem of stuttering for someone who has a history of psychological problems can be successfully managed without extensive psychotherapeutic treatment for those problems. Louise had an extensive history of family and marital conflicts, yet she managed to achieve a satisfactory solution for the stuttering.

We believe that her success in gaining control over the overt features of the stuttering was a crucial factor and doubtless had a great deal of psychotherapeutic value. We viewed Louise as someone who felt that she had never had much control over what happened to her along the way; however, and we believe this was another important factor in this success story, she seldom indulged in self-pity. The control she achieved over the stuttering behavior gave her confidence, we think, to believe she could exercise control over her life in other ways. The control also had another benefit of considerable significance. It helped to resolve her feelings of ugliness. Combined with the change in her feelings about her teeth, it served to solve an important self-concept problem.

The achievement of the successful control illustrates something else about successful therapy. Although it can sometimes be a function of a single technique or of some uniquely profound experience, it is usually a function of the effects of a combination of interrelated circumstances and experiences. In this case, for example, we believe the initial favorable circumstance was the time of the treatment. Louise came for help at a time when doing something about her stuttering was probably more necessary than at any other time in her life. Next, the group experience did a great deal for the morale of this case and facilitated confidence in the treatment approach. The experience with Wendell Johnson's book was another significant factor. Perhaps it served to ameliorate her guilt feelings, since a major theme of that book is that stuttering is created by parental misinterpretations and the erroneous labeling of normal fluency in children as stuttering. It relieves the stutterer of any responsibility as the source of his problem. Or perhaps the contents somehow tied things together at a time when Louise was trying to combine information into meaningful ideas. We cannot be certain, but in any case the book provided a profound experience that served as an important element of the ultimate success. Finally, there was the environmental change. We seriously doubt that Louise would have become an example of a clinical success if she had remained in the old environment. The new environment made it more possible for her to work to consolidate the changed attitudes and the control over her stuttering.

The environmental shift and the favorable experiences that

Louise had in the new environment illustrate one other feature of therapy that may determine success or failure. It is the element of luck. We believe Louise had good luck. She seemed to have gotten the job that was just right for her. She got the right man. She had a successful experience with a relapse. Everything turned out well. We cannot know how things might have turned out if she had gotten a different job, or a different man, or had not been able to recover from the relapse. Moreover, if she had not had relatives in that community who made it possible for her to effect the change, she could not have gone there at all. We do believe there is an element of luck in many clinical successes, and that this case illustrates how it can be a part of a successful therapy experience.

A CLINICAL FAILURE: HARRY
CLINICIAN: FRANK B. ROBINSON

Harry impressed us favorably immediately. He was 24 years old, tall, well built, and handsome. He wore a two hundred dollar suit and had social manners that we imagined were customary evidence of an association with an Ivy League University and a family background of wealth and high social status. He was loquacious, affable, urbane, intelligent, and we were certain, a person of good character.

The overt stuttering he presented was of a relatively mild form consisting of two or three quick repetitions of word elements or, occasionally, brief fixations of articulatory postures accompanied by slight tremors. However, these signs of a stuttering problem were not evident frequently. He was admittedly clever at substitution and other verbal manipulations. Thus, he usually gave the impression of a person who stuttered only occasionally. He reported having many acquaintances and a few good friends who he was certain didn't know he was a stutterer. But he said his stuttering bothered him a great deal. It was very embarrassing, and he was always under a lot of tension and strain.

When he read aloud, the "sticky" blocks were more frequent and somewhat more pronounced and his embarrassment was obvious. Yet the overt stuttering certainly wasn't severe, and as we talked with him we felt that treatment would be relatively easy, particularly after we explained our treatment approach and emphasized the importance of having him test the validity of his concern about the stuttering by stuttering openly and freely. He thought it would be very difficult, but he expressed a determination to do anything necessary (he was planning to become a stockbroker, and "I've got to do something about this stuttering.") and proceeded to demonstrate his willingness by making a telephone call on which he deliberately faked stuttering on two words. His courage was something else we liked about this person.

From his autobiography and the initial interviews we learned much about Harry that, of course, should have warned us. His life story revealed obvious evidence of marked and persistent family conflicts and presented a picture of a very sensitive over-indulged person who had never been able to experience satisfactory identification with either parent. The father was a self-made man who had achieved early success as an industrialist and inventor and who then had married a woman who came from a wealthy and prominent family. Unfortunately, the mother was ignorant about cooking and housekeeping and child-rearing. The most vivid impression Harry had of his parents was the arguing they did over the way the house was kept and the way the four children were allowed to behave. His mother would retreat to a back bedroom. His father would escape to his club where he would sometimes stay for a week. Harry thought his parents probably would have been divorced if it had not been for their religion.

His account of school years revealed a consistent picture of compensatory behavior. He was always becoming involved in some extra-curricular activity. He was a good athlete and would let his studies go to be in a tournament. He played tennis; he was an expert with guns; he had trophies for fishing tournaments in Mexico and Jamaica. In high school he was involved with the school annual and also had operated an investment club. He got by with mediocre grades until he went to college. There his propensity for extra-curricular activities created greater academic problems. He still had not graduated when he came to the clinic. He said he planned to return after he got established in business which he thought he could do in a year or two. Meanwhile, he would stay at home ("as long as I can stand it") and he had expense money from an inheritance.

He told his story well. We noted certain signs of hostility, of marked feelings of insecurity, of guilt, and of immature behavior. And normally we doubtless would have been quite guarded in our prognosis. But we were dazzled and beguiled, we know now, by the aura of wealth and sophistication surrounding this case. There was a definite halo effect. We wanted to help this fellow (cultivate is what we really had in mind), and we ignored the danger signs.

We arranged to work with Harry individually three one hour sessions weekly. It is doubtless significant to the story of this failure that the sessions usually extended to an hour and a half or even two hours.

He was a good listener as well as a good talker. We enjoyed his company. And the therapy was very successful at first. He tackled the problem of his sensitivity about stuttering with gusto. We went on projects together and took turns stuttering and exploring the listeners' reactions. We had many interesting discussions about stuttering.

Identification with the therapist occurred quickly. Of course, identification of the therapist with the case had already occurred.

Harry lost his feelings of embarrassment about his stuttering rapidly. And with that change he lost much of his stuttering. We worked at helping him learn how to control the occasional blocks he had. Everything went along fine. We discussed the possibility of relapse and reactions to it. During that time, which was well along in the second month, and in the context of possible relapse, there were discussions of his family situation and his future in general. But by this time, the discussions were more like conversations between two good friends. Most of these occurred in the campus coffee shop, and two were held in a plush club where he had invited us to meet some of his friends, and where, of course, we were pleased to go.

Then, during a period of two or three weeks he appeared, each time we met, to be having greater difficulty with his speech. The sticky blocks were back and some of the repetitious pattern. He still talked glowingly about how things were going. He could tell us nothing that might explain the relapse. We now began to appreciate the trap we were in. The relationship we had developed with this case prevented him from admitting any problems that might place him in an unfavorable light. He could not tolerate an adverse change in the image we had given him of himself. We could not now be a clinician for anything but the stuttering behavior. We continued trying to help him re-establish the former controls with the stuttering behavior, but with little success. We also continued to question him about circumstances at home and at his work, but here too we had no real success. The sessions became increasingly strained and awkward. He began to be late and sometimes he would telephone and leave word that he could not come. Finally, he stopped coming altogether.

Some time later we learned what had happened from a mutual friend. First, his business experience had not been successful. About the time he stopped coming to the clinic he had dropped that project and had begun to take charge of the political campaign for a mayorality candidate. Second, he had had a quarrel with his father and moved to an apartment and was having difficulty supporting himself. The informant said that Harry was currently trying to get his father to provide the financial support for his campaigning project.

What did we learn from this? For one thing, we had had a vivid experience with a particular kind of clinical error that may frequently be made by students in the course of their training, but not by the experienced professional therapist. We refer to the friendship that was established early with this case and which dominated the relationship. Although an element of friendliness is an important ingredient of any successful clinical relationship, it does not follow that success in being perceived by a client as a friendly person signifies effective therapy. Moreover, a friendly relationship that includes accepting invitations to be entertained socially by a client may be permissible when therapy has been successfully concluded, but it can never serve as an appropriate foundation for the interaction required for effective treatment.

However, the friendly relationship was by no means the most important factor in this particular example of a clinical failure.

Much more critical was the reason for the cultivation of Harry's friendship. We completely failed to recognize a personal need to identify with the class of people that Harry appeared to us to personify. Our lack of insight was an appalling truth. We had exploited this case for our personal benefit. And in so doing, we fostered a kind of relationship that permitted Harry to continue to use the facade of his social sophistication to cover a host of problems, and it was too late when we realized that the stuttering in this case was intricately interrelated with other personal problems. We shall not soon forget our experience with Harry.

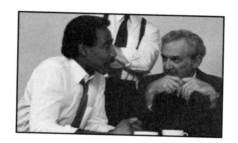

A CLINICAL SUCCESS: LEONARD
CLINICIAN: JOSEPH SHEEHAN

Leonard was both one of the severest stutterers that I have ever encountered and one of the most normal and healthy in personality. Since we have now known him for over eighteen years, we have an excellent followup on his progress and on the outcome of his therapy.

The effect of stuttering on the personality is frequently not as great as might be assumed for, despite the severity of his handicap, Leonard had an easy outgoing personality and was a clinically normal adult. Considering his communication problems, he had developed astonishing social facility.

Leonard was waiting for me when I arrived at UCLA as a new member of the faculty. He had undergone some abortive therapy in the public schools in California around the fifth or sixth grade and had gone through a summer speech improvement camp experience in the Midwest. He had come to UCLA to try the Dunlap approach and had begun some training in negative practice with Drs. George Lehner and Maxine Gunderson. When I first met Leonard he was still trying to imitate his own stuttering a la Dunlap, but it was not a close duplication of his true pattern.

Leonard's habitual pattern consisted of a violent tilting back of his head; rolling his eyes toward the ceiling; the muscles in his neck would stand out; he would become flushed; he would twist his face in a forced grimace; attempt various starters; some head jerks in an effort to release himself from the block; and also would accompany his stuttering with various bodily gestures. He had little fluency capacity and stuttered severely on almost every word. His name and words beginning with the same sound as his first and last names were especially difficult.

He had so often distended and flexed his neck muscles during his blocks that he wore a large collar size for his weight. Later, as he reduced his struggling behavior during stuttering, he was able to reduce his collar size as well—a nice operational definition of his return to normality. But much happened before then. We return now to Leonard as a bull-necked struggler with words.

Leonard was one of two brothers who stuttered. His older brother had begun stuttering at the age of six, at the time Leonard was born—a significant precursor of their relationship. Leonard himself began stuttering at about the age of three and became considerably more severe than his brother. Although there were moments of closeness between the brothers as they grew up, there was always a heavy undercurrent of rivalry. In fact, when I first began to work with Leonard, his brother was being treated psychoanalytically by Dr. Lee Travis. Thus Leonard and his brother were not only rivals but had gone to therapists who were in themselves professional siblings in southern California! During the course of their therapies they would argue occasionally about who was following the right approach.

Leonard reported that his stuttering began with repetitions and with blockings. The stuttering had first been noticed by his mother and father about the age of three, although teachers had played an important part in his first vivid stuttering experience. This occurred when he was about six, when he was placed in a speech class, where he first remembers blocking severely. He felt startled at the amount of difficulty.

Leonard had lived in Detroit until the age of 13 when his family moved to southern California. His father was in the wholesale fish business during his early years and later a real estate broker. He relates, "My father was uninvolved with the family and with me except with money." Leonard's mother was sometimes accepting, sometimes entirely rejecting. She had told him that if he was going to stutter, he shouldn't speak at all. When he did stutter, a hurt look came over her face.

Leonard felt that his brother was always preferred, that he was more rejected than the brother. Thus, Leonard began stuttering at the age of three in a family in which, within his memory, a preferred nine-year-old brother had always stuttered. A symptom of protest? A bid for attention? Identification with a more successful rival? While we cannot be sure looking backward, any one of these seemed a possible pathway to stuttering for Leonard, and his brother remained for years a most important figure in Leonard's life. Now that Leonard has found himself and a new style and ease in speaking, his brother has melted more appropriately into the background of Leonard's life.

Soon after he entered the clinic, Lenoard took our intake battery which in his case consisted of a Rorschach, TAT, DAP, MMPI, LOA, and a history. The results revealed many positive personality assets, including good quality M or Movement responses on the Rorschach. Leonard's group was included in the Rorschach prognostic study which we undertook in the early 1950's, and Leonard's improvement was in line with the findings on the prognostic potential of the Rorschach. He was also included in our LOA (Level of Aspiration) study and showed higher self-esteem and less defensiveness than most stutterers included in that study.

Leonard was in therapy at the UCLA clinic from 1949 to 1953, again for a brief period in 1956, and much later, following two years of individual psychotherapy, he returned for "finishing touches" in 1965. Upon his return in 1965, Leonard spent half his time in the clinic working on his own speech; the balance of the time, he began to assume the role of auxiliary therapist to the new stutterers coming into the clinic. This experience has proved especially significant to him and partially accounts for his more complete recovery.

Now to the therapy itself. Suttering was viewed as an approach-avoidance conflict, as a form of learned behavior, and the basic goal of therapy was the reduction of all tendencies to avoidance, whatever the source. This approach is covered partially in two articles by Sheehan, *J. Psychology*, 1953, and *JSHD*, 1954, on presentation of a conflict theory and integration of psychotherapy with speech therapy. The Speech Foundation booklet, *On Stuttering and It's Treatment*, contains numerous examples of the therapy in operation.

Leonard worked both individually and in a succession of therapy groups. He had contact both with each new group and with various advanced groups that were formed during his time in the clinic. Always he was one of the most courageous. Leonard would try anything, though never in a reckless or foolhardy fashion. He possessed both discernment enough to see what needed to be done and guts enough to do it—a happy combination for a stutterer. He had a kind of stubbornness or dogged persistence that he was able to turn into an asset in therapy. For many stutterers stubbornness is a liability!

Among specific techniques he worked on were these: keeping eye contact while stuttering; freely accepting the role of stutterer; openly discussing stuttering; observing closely what he did when he stuttered; monitoring visually via mirror work, aurally via recordings, tactually as he trained himself to feel how he stuttered; making a block longer in order to make it easier; resisting audience rejection, time pressure, interruption threat; stuttering voluntarily on non-feared words with varying patterns; stuttering openly and forward as possible on feared words; observation of the fact that he spoke many words normally and fluently; self-observation aimed to demonstrate that his stuttering was not something that happened to him, but something that he did, his own behavior; stuttering as easily as possible; constantly expanding the circle of situation difficulty entered; continuing open discussion of stuttering and frequent identification of himself as a person who stuttered.

Among further methods, Leonard would practice: stuttering without one of his major tricks; adaptation to delayed speech feedback; creating especially difficult and challenging speaking situations; assuming responsibility for his own speech behavior; and overcoming avoidances at every level.

For example, he would sit on the steps of the Psychology building at UCLA, reading aloud the Daily Bruin, stuttering freely and openly to all passersby in the process. He would ask questions of bus drivers at intersections, just as the light changed and they were about to take off. He learned to resist time pressures from others, and to cease putting himself into the built-in time pressure system to which nearly every stutterer constantly subjects himself.

The aim of reducing avoidance for the sake of future improvement was constantly stressed—at first briefly to Leonard, then by him to himself and other stutterers. As Leonard began to assume the role of auxiliary clinician, he did a significantly better job on his own speech.

Leonard attributes his greatest improvement to the period 1950-52, which coincides with our own observations and to the observer evaluations made during that period in the Rorschach prognosis study.

Throughout the early part of his therapy in the clinic, Leonard continued to work on the Dunlap method, attempting an exact duplication of his true stuttering pattern as a means of changing the habitual pattern. Research we conducted in the 1950's comparing the effects of the Dunlap technique, a bounce technique, and a slide or smooth prolongation as means of voluntarily stuttering (Sheehan, *JSHD*, 1957), added to our growing disillusionment with the initiation of the true pattern. Leonard shifted to a still greater emphasis on the reduction of avoidance and the strengthening of approach behaviors. Since the experiment showed that the Dunlap technique did more harm than good, it is interesting that Leonard improved during the 1950-52 period in spite of using it part of the time. But he was doing many other things of greater importance all in the direction of reducing avoidance and developing an easier and more open way of stuttering.

Our experience with Leonard and negative practice illustrates an important principle in stuttering therapy, *i.e.*, a mistake in technique can be absorbed successfully provided the total relationship is good and provided the individual has enough personality assets to move forward despite flaws in the therapy.

Leonard's social adjustment had always been more than adequate, and he had enjoyed a normal dating life. In 1953 occurred an event which we wish we could arrange for all our stutterers, for its major effects appear definitely therapeutic. Leonard married an attractive girl who had come from the Midwest to study speech therapy and psychology. The marriage has turned out satisfying, to use Leonard's term, and appeared to consolidate the gains Leonard had already made through the combination of stuttering therapy and psychotherapy just summarized.

For two years prior to returning to the clinic for finishing touches in 1965, Leonard had two years of psychotherapy. While he did not make any actual improvement on his stuttering during that time, he feels that greater awareness of his feelings helped him to preserve gains already made and enabled him to continue improvement. Upon returning, he spent part of the time working in an advanced group on his own speech and part of the time as a beginner's group co-therapist. He has profited from both roles and speaks with much greater smoothness now.

At present Leonard is working as a geophysicist, has a daughter 11 and a son 9, is still happily married, and appears to have found fulfillment in life. Avocationally, he continues to function as an auxiliary member of the clinic staff, and he is one of our most effective speech clinicians. He is perceptive and makes incisive analyses of the tricks and avoidance mechanisms used by each new group of stutterers, and he is respected by them all. While he still has some moments of hesitation and choppiness in his speech, he is continuing to work and to improve, and he is usually within the normal range of fluency. He now enjoys himself as a speaker and takes pride in his new ability. Leonard is his real name, and his self-acceptance is such that he has approved the use of it.

A CLINICAL FAILURE: RUDOLF
CLINICIAN: JOSEPH SHEEHAN

The case of Rudolf illustrates well that while the therapeutic relationship is important, and while motivation is important, the outcome is not always exclusively within the grasp of the participants in therapy. This case illustrates the crucial role of timing in the evaluation of results. Followup and timing of evaluation are of such central significance that today's apparent success may become tomorrow's failure, while today's failure may turn out successfully in the long run. This failure case, Rudolf, could at one stage have been labelled a success. Possibly, in the future, he could still become one.

Rudolf was a 16-year-old German boy who was referred to us by a famous midwestern medical clinic. On the referral it was noted that members of the Neurology section of the clinic who had seen Rudolf had mentioned that there was some indication of emotional disturbance. However, because of the attitude of the parents, they recommended that speech therapy be tried first to see whether an improvement in speaking would not result in Rudolf's being able to handle emotional difficulties without psychiatric help. A tic was also noted at the medical clinic.

Rudolf was the only son of a high-placed member of the German business community in the United States. Rudolf's entrance through our door was a most vivid and memorable occasion.

The lad was ushered into the room by his father who rather stiffly introduced himself with a thick German accent and a heavy sweep of authority, bowing quickly with military bearing. Rudolf pulled himself awkwardly into a rigid stance of *achtung*, clumped his heels together, and crouched beatenly in a very low bow to acknowledge the introduction. His father grunted with evident satisfaction at Rudolf's performance, and we gathered that the boy had met the test this time. Later we would confirm what we then suspected, that Rudolf was striving to get away from such rituals. He had been in this country two years and was attending a Los Angeles public high school.

Rudolf himself was a reddish-blond, awkwardly coltish lad who came in as an extremely severe stutterer with many bodily movements and facial grimaces. He had little apparent fluency capacity and blocked severely on nearly every word. In addition, at periods of greater tension, Rudolf suffered from a tic, consisting in a spasmodic tilting of his head. What made Rudolf tic? It was inviting to speculate the possible relationship between the boy's head-tilting tic and his father's insistence on subservience to authority. While the tic sometimes occurred during moments of stuttering, it also tended to occur without speech during periods of heightened tension. These typically occurred more at home and on vactions than at school and appeared to be related to fear of the father. The tic never appeared in the therapy sessions following the first one. When Rudolf came to therapy he would drop the tic as soon as he came in the door.

Among his other problems, Rudolf had a lateral lisp which he recalled had affected him in his native German as well.

Our therapy with Rudolf was a combination of psychotherapy and speech therapy relating to his stuttering and tic and articulation therapy relating to his lateral lisp. Another speech therapist worked with Rudolf on his lisp and assisted with some aspects of the stuttering therapy.

We viewed the members of the family as members of the problem and undertook a form of family therapy. For example, we held discussions with Rudolf's parents in an effort to reduce the severity of discipline, the stress on absolute obedience, and pressures for school achievement. While the mother was willing to soften things for Rudolf, the father was stiff-backed, stubborn, and essentially unyielding, though he obviously considered himself eager to cooperate and said so. We pointed out that Rudolf was showing danger signals and that their contined insistence on holding him to rigid standards in the face of these signals represented a kind of incorrigibility on their part. Though the mother had for years provided support, she too was afraid of the father—physically afraid. Rudolf later confided that his father had hit both of them and that they were afraid of him.

To understand the pattern of this family, we administered psychological test batteries to all three. Both parents showed essentially normal MMPI profiles and were more intelligent and better adjusted than Rudolf. On the basis of Rorschach, TAT, DAP, and MMPI results, Rudolf emerged as a fairly disturbed young man. He showed the MMPI's "neurotic triad," appeared to feel rebellious toward authority, and revealed some loosening of reality ties. Dependency, hostility, and passivity were prominent features of his dynamics along with an identification with the aggressor, braggadocio tendencies, and a contempt for weakness. For example, women were seen as weak and, therefore, worthy of contempt—ironic in view of his mother's supportive attitude—but Rudolf had taken on his feared father's values.

Rudolf's feelings about himself as well as about school are well caught up in one of his TAT stories, 17 BM, in which there is a man climbing a rope. He described the fellow as "one of those underachievers, they don't feel secure, they always have to brag to cover up . . . Suddenly the rope is going to break, and he will fall down and get a broken leg." He entitled this picture, "The Bragger."

The onset of Rudolf's stuttering was obscured in the mists of vague parental recall, yet it appeared to have developed around age three. At that time, the father, a former member of Hitler's SS elite corps, deserted home for a year. The stuttering which began during this period continued after the father's return.

Rudolf was afraid not only of parental authority in a general psychological sense but had a specific physical fear of his father. It was a long time in therapy before he became comfortable enough to be able to talk about his father—when he did, the tic reappeared though it had been absent from therapy sessions. At first, Rudolf talked about what a great fellow the father was—a sort of Teutonic Superman. Only later was he able to confide his fears and smouldering resentments.

Though he was almost a World War I movie stereotype of a Prussian military figure, Rudolf's father was uniformly pleasant with an attitude of eager cooperation. He appeared to see what we were driving at in terms of his contribution to the boy's problem, but he was unable to do much more than experience it as a failure in himself. Moreover, he was pervasively ashamed of Rudolf. The boy was a disappointment and a threat to him. He acted as though the mother had brought some kind of weakness into the family. Rudolf knew his father was ashamed of him and in turn felt more demoralized. The father had attempted to use "discipline"—military, Prussian discipline—as a means of straightening Rudolf out, but the boy didn't have much ramrod about him.

Rudolf's relationship with his mother was much more positive —a good relationship. Though there was no great warmth, especially on his part toward her, it was still his best relationship. Interestingly, he had adopted the German attitude toward women—they were inferior, belonged only in the home, etc. His mother was indeed weak and inferior in the only home Rudolf knew.

Everything German was good and to be preserved. The servants were German, and German was spoken in the home. Rudolf's life was regimented down to the last detail—what to eat, what clothes to wear, what language to use when, how to be courteous and to whom, etc. Rudolf came to resent all these things and didn't even want to talk in German to his family. He was beginning to like America; even worse, Rudolf was beginning to become Americanized. As he did so, he progressed on his speech and his tic disappeared.

Along with providing emotional support and opportunity for discussion of his feelings, the therapy with Rudolf was oriented toward action—carrying out of assignments within the limits of his ability to fulfill them successfully. We worked on self-confrontation with the stuttering behavior itself, with eye contact during moments of stuttering, with speaking and stuttering more freely and openly, with discussion assignments, voluntary stuttering in different styles, showing him how to stutter in a new and easier way—in short, we tried to provide for Rudolf many of the kinds of basic experiences proved most helpful with stutterers.

The philosophy and many examples of the approach to stuttering therapy employed here has been described in Sheehan's chapter, "Conflict Theory of Stuttering," in the Eisenson symposium and in two booklets published by the Speech Foundation of America: (1) *On Stuttering and Its Treatment;* (2) *Treatment of the Young Stutterer.* Though we studied carefully the background of Rudolf's problem and tried to change his environment by reducing parental pressures, the emphasis was on action, on the performance of assignments. He learned in time to formulate some of these himself and was able to succeed more often than he failed.

Rudolf's response to the therapy and to the assignments was generally positive and frequently enthusiastic. He did become much more open, stopped avoiding words, talked more openly about himself and his stuttering. And he improved, not suddenly but dramatically, over the period of ten months of therapy. By the ninth month, he was speaking fluently most of the time and stuttering calmly and easily when he did have trouble. His tic had entirely disappeared. He had corrected his lateral lisp and and found a new pride in speaking and in himself.

How then can Rudolf be considered a failure? Had we made the assessment at nine months of therapy Rudolf would have been considered a success worth raving about. Startling indeed had been the changes, especially to anyone who had not seen him during the period of the therapy. How did an apparent clinical success become a failure?

Enter the father. The Americanization of Rudolf, he suddenly decided, had gone far enough. The boy had been attending "inferior" US schools for three years. He was finding new freedom along with new fluency and was growing rebellious. His father did not like Rudolf's associations nor how he was turning out. Without in any way consulting us the father made arrangements for Rudolf to attend a boarding school back in Germany in a town and place strange to him. He would know no one, for his mother and father were staying here.

As he related this development, Rudolf stated repeatedly that he was happy, for now he was going back to Germany. He had been told, "You're going to enjoy this." After nearly an hour of a somewhat swaggering buildup on the glories of Germany and the extent of his happiness over going back, Rudolf suddenly revealed how scared he was. He began to worry about his speech, about how far behind he would be in Latin, Math, etc., since U.S. schools were "inferior." He offered himself reassurance pointing out a little forlornly that he could visit his grandmother.

As tension related to his going back to Germany built up on Rudolf, his speech began to show signs of breaking down, and then the tic came back. There was however no regression on the laterial lisp. Rudolf had been proud of having worked on his speech, of having worked hard. He had been doing better in school and his grades had improved. His attitude toward U.S. schools now was that they weren't preparing him adequately; at the same time, this was a face-saving device for failing gracefully if he encountered trouble in school in Germany as he had in the past.

Rudolf's father requested that we send a report to a German M.D. whom he had chosen to conduct any further treatment the young man might need. Even if we had been consulted we would have found it difficult to recommend anyone in Rudolf's vicinity, but we did not get the chance. We prepared the report and sent it to the German physician, who to our knowledge had no special familiarity with *Das Stottern*, but received no acknowledgment. Upon further request and as an experiment in parental confrontation therapy, we also sent a copy to Rudolf's father and mother. Nothing more from them. Truth is a dubious route to popularity.

Somewhere in Germany a reddish-blond young man tilts his head jerkily and grimaces as he speaks, perhaps awaiting the day when he can throw off the yoke of discipline, find himself, and become his own authority.

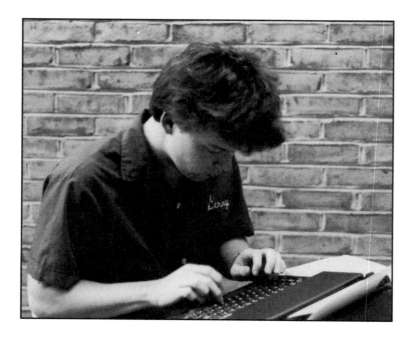

A CLINICAL SUCCESS: ALEX
CLINICIAN: ALASTAIR A. STUNDEN

Alex came to the clinic for the express purpose of eliminating his stuttering. He was referred by a speech therapist who was familiar with the work of the clinic and who had treated Alex on several occasions for periods up to a year. According to Alex's report, this therapist had not been able to finish the job.

Alex's history was somewhat atypical in the sense that he did not remember stuttering until his teens. His preteen period he felt was fluent with no speech problems of any kind. This issue continued to puzzle him and even after therapy he never really understood why his stuttering had developed at all. His most easily recalled memory about stuttering was his feeling of resentment at his inability to move easily with his fellows in the social life of his school and community.

As he remembered it, his stuttering was marked by wide fluctuations. He believed his fluent periods were directly related to his work with his speech therapist, but he was at a complete loss to account for his consistent relapses despite the fact that these events were consistently correlated with obvious environmental stress such as the taking of examinations at the university, moving from one community to another, and so on. Interestingly enough, it was at these times he would cut off his relationship with his therapist, frequently for practical reasons associated with the environmental demand.

Alex's family was composed of his father, a respected and well liked automobile mechanic; his mother, a weak woman, easily dominated by the family; a brother, several years younger; and a baby sister, born when Alex was 19 years old.

Alex talked little in a spontaneous way about his family during the course of the treatment period and not much became known of his feelings about them except for some pleasant memories of visits to the country.

Alex was 22 years old when he arrived at the clinic, and he had just completed a degree in business administration. He was tall, somewhat gangly but handsome, well-mannered, a careful dresser, and a severe stutterer. He impressed everyone with his friendliness and openness despite his extraordinary difficulty in communicating. When talking his eyes would roll, his neck would stretch, his voice would strain, break and finally screech into a gravelly falsetto. All of this was accompanied by awkward postures that required the listener to back away for fear Alex might suddenly flail out with an arm or foot.

In social relationships, Alex appeared quite comfortable. He quickly established his own contacts at the university and did not rely, as did some of the other patients, on the obvious, quasi-therapeutic relationships available within the framework of the clinic.

On interview one was continually impressed with his lack of overt anxiety and demonstrable ego strength that took the form of accepting any challenge issued to him despite the difficulty level as long as it was clearly related to working on his speech.

Alex was a member of a group of patients all of whom had come some distance and made some personal sacrifice to spend the intensive year of speech therapy that made up the clinic program. Each patient was in therapy four days a week for two to three hours per day. The routine of therapy followed the pattern of group meeting with the therapist followed by individual contacts with student clinicians. The therapy itself also followed traditional lines, focusing on a set of successive approximations each dependent on what had gone before, designed to eliminate all attempts to avoid stuttering. A second goal was to modify the stuttering behavior so that efforts at communication were more rewarding. The final step in therapy was the preparation of the patient for fluency and the acceptance of himself as a reasonable fluent speaker.

The cardinal rule in this therapeutic procedure was the elimination of all avoidance. None of the group members was to tolerate any withholding of stuttering behavior. Everyone was to stutter until he reached the point at which stuttering, if it was to occur at all, had to be done voluntarily with conscious effort. Fear reduction was the underlying theoretical theme and feared words, situations, and relationships were sought out and explored until the fear was exhausted. Clearly it was assumed by the therapist that the group members, Alex included, were suffering from the kind of stuttering that was a reaction to their unsuccessful attempts to edit out previously punished, hence fear-producing, motor speech behaviors.

Alex's progress during the course of this therapy was not particularly surprising. He soon gave up his posturings and his falsetto squeaks were quickly forgotten. Thus, his stuttering became real in the sense that he no longer engaged in behaviors which aided him in the avoidance of non-fluencies, but he was now actively and openly non-fluent. His speech began to approximate that of the normal speaker with the exception of a few more hesitations and repetitions than might otherwise be typical of normal speech. Alex was getting better.

Alex's behavior in the group was that of a cooperative participant interested only in carrying out the next assignment. That the assignment led to further success only reinforced his basic belief that he was at last, after several failures, on the right track. And well he might be after 3,000 miles of travel and a significant interruption in his career goals. In truth, Alex found himself in the unenviable position of having to adjust his long-standing magical beliefs about the wondrous advances of "University Brand Speech Pathology" to the reality of a relatively routine therapeutic situation virtually parallel to those he had previously experienced. This was further complicated by the fact that the therapist who had interviewed him and with whom Alex thought he was going to work had left to take a similar position at another university clinic. It soon became apparent that these factors were beginning to influence Alex's response to therapy.

As best as it can be pieced together, he began to see it in this way. First of all he had made the commitment to come to therapy 3,000 miles from home. He felt under an obligation to follow it through, and his initial responses to the therapy and the therapist were made in that framework. Alex believed, in effect, that it was necessary for him to profit from this experience, and his behavior was consonant with that felt goal. Secondly, and most important, Alex began to improve. But here he was not without his history, a history of working with a speech therapist, getting better and then relapsing. As was indicated earlier, the phenomena associated with the relapses were never really accessible to him and the nature of the therapy conducted at the clinic precluded the kind of exploration that might have uncovered significant information related to these experiences. Thus, about half-way through the year, Alex's belief in his commitment to therapy began to be overtaken by his now equally strong belief that he had once more gotten himself into therapy only to fail. That this might really be his feeling became apparent when he started passively refusing to perform his assignments. He also began to subvert openly the activities of the other group members by punishing severely any of their failures and encouraging a kind of laissez-faire attitude toward therapy. At the same time, Alex began to express loudly his uncertainty about his own success and his tacit lack of faith in the therapist by questioning the validity of the therapist's therapy. The group was stunned and the therapist dismayed. The one member whose success in therapy was patent to all who had known him at the beginning of the year was leading a revolt.

During a particularly distressing interchange with Alex while in one of the group sessions, it became obvious I would have to do something. What I wanted to do was to restore Alex's belief in the therapy (therapist) and, at the same time, his belief in himself. The solution was immediate, and I presented it to him in the midst of our discussion. Might it not be possible to restore Alex's faith in his ability to profit from the therapy by giving him assignments designed to precipitate his predictable relapse?

Alex was offered the challenge, and he accepted it. His task was to carry out the assignments of the therapy in reverse. That is, instead of giving up all avoidances he was to reinstitute them. Even more, he was to seek them out, make them up, take every opportunity to avoid normal speech attempts and escape from fluency. He was given hand movements to perform as release devices. He was given the assignment of leaving the room when the telephone rang regardless of the situation and so on. The suggestion was also offered that if he carried out the assignments successfully he would be unable to speak at all within ten days. It took only seven.

Alex ended the year a comfortable stutterer. He was comfortable with himself, with his residual stuttering, and with his new found ability to assume the responsibility for his own behavior. In discussions afterwards it came out that in all his previous experiences with fluency he had never felt responsible for getting there. Somehow it had always been something that had been done *to* him rather than *by* him. Further, Alex had never really grasped the important therapeutic principle that we are our problem. Not only did he feel no responsibility for his fluency, but he also felt no responsibility for his stuttering. In every way, stuttering for him was something that just happened to him over which he had no control. That he was able to direct and influence his stuttering was amazing to him. The therapist's decision to precipitate the relapse resulted in a dramatic and significant insight.

Alex also became aware of the fact that to be successful in therapy he had to really become something different. It was not possible for him to return to his pre-therapy existence if he were to maintain the changes he had created. He recognized too that it was possible for him to begin deciding how much change he wanted to make. He no longer made the demand that he be cured of stuttering. He was willing to accept himself for what he was with the firm knowledge that it was his choice.

A CLINICAL FAILURE: ARTHUR
CLINICIAN: ALASTAIR A. STUNDEN

Arthur had come from Michigan. He arrived, 21 years old and newly graduated, with all his possessions piled into his bright red Volkswagen. He was tall, well-muscled, almost handsome, with eyes a bit too far apart to fit well with the rest of his features. He came to the clinic after an extensive exploration of the other programs in the country. He had written letters, talked with various professionals and read all the books. He was convinced that *if* anyone could help him, we could.

Arthur's memories of his early experiences with stuttering always remained vague while in treatment at the clinic. From all he could piece together he had begun to stutter severely about the age of five after a fight with another kid. It was difficult for him to remember himself as never having stuttered, and he felt that his stuttering, even in his early years, was about as severe as it was when he came to the clinic. He had had treatment ranging from work in the public schools to therapy in the college speech clinic in his home town with a stop or two along the way at offices of psychiatrists. His stuttering had always made life difficult for him, but he typically reacted to these experiences by working even harder to overcome any handicap his stuttering created. Courage in the face of impossible odds was a good description of his orientation to himself and this maxim was to contribute in an important way to his progress in therapy.

Arthur was a graduate of a major mid-western university, had played varsity football and basketball, lettered in track, swimming and golf, and during summer vacations had worked as a stevedore. He majored in philosophy, graduated *cum laude* and his ambition after completing a Master's degree was to write and teach. He was engaged to an attractive girl he had met in college, and it was on her income that he planned to live while finishing his graduate degree.

Arthur's family was composed of his father and namesake, a structural engineer; his mother, a housewife who died after a protracted illness when Arthur was 15 years old; and a married sister, two years younger than Arthur. The most significant member of the family was Arthur's father whose arbitrary and oftentimes sadistic responses to his wife and children were a constant source of upset and irritation. Arthur frequently found himself in the position of having to defend himself for behavior which in other families would never be challenged. For example, Arthur's father was very much concerned about personal cleanliness and would frequently supervise the bathing habits of the entire family. That Arthur may have adequately performed this task without the direct supervision of his father was of no consequence if it was suddenly decided that a bath was in order. Another example of his father's sadistic attitude had to do with family members being on time. Arthur's father ate meals, dressed, went to bed and relaxed by the clock. To be late to dinner meant no dinner and a vicious, degrading lecture in front of family or guests. Arthur would occasionally attempt to defend himself or his sister and would receive an even stronger tongue lashing for interfering with his father's obsessive preoccupation with time. Further, it was not possible for Arthur to play freely with his friends unless he was prepared to run two gauntlets. The first had to do with his father insisting on elaborate cleansing procedures designed more to implant in his son a morbid fear of illness than to ensure good personal hygiene. The second related to the factor of time. To get home from play with sufficient latitude to ensure prompt completion of the necessary washing rituals was very hard for a young boy to do.

Some of the things that Arthur learned from this relationship was that male authority figures were inconsistent, unreliable, arbitrary, devious, inconsiderate, uninterested, and most important, likely to have a hidden agenda that would result in Arthur's being punished. He also learned that when confronted by male figures his best recourse was to keep quiet.

Arthur's stuttering was a source of genuine concern for the family, his father included. However, very early Arthur learned that he and his stuttering were separate events that could be reacted to by others as if they were independent of each other. For example, his father did not attempt to impose temporal restrictions on Arthur's stuttering behavior. Attempts were made by the family members to relieve Arthur's discomfort about talking by talking for him. This procedure only served to irritate him and make him feel more under the control of his family than ever. He seemed to recognize intuitively that if he ever gave in to the abject terror he felt most of the time by failing to fight back his chances for psychological survival were very remote.

This obvious relationship between his stuttering and his interaction with his father was never explored by Arthur during the course of therapy. (Arthur, like Alex, was a member of a group of stutterers who met four times a week for three hours per day. The group members met with the therapist for one hour and later met individually with student clinicians.) It was my feeling that these data were psychologically inaccessible because of the threat that was related to them. Furthermore, within the group, Arthur was unable (or did not want to) discuss any kind of feeling and soon found himself a peripheral member because of his constant denial of feeling states as a factor in his stuttering. The alternatives to this hypothesis, and it was the one that was maintained by Arthur in his occasional individual conferences with me, was that there was no longer any significance to be found in examining this relationship because he was now responsible for his own behavior and was more than capable of adequate self direction.

As a stutterer Arthur was very severe. Any conversation with him was an extraordinary experience in frustration and discomfort for both the listener and Arthur. Even his simplest and most insignificant comments were rapidly reduced to endless, painful periods that were often terminated before the communication was complete with a fluent "You know" or "Oh well." He gave no evidence of having any ability to establish easy, comfortable relationships with people but was constantly presenting a picture to others of serious, politely anxious solemnity that bordered on the ludicrous. He was never spontaneous, usually holding back all speech attempts until it was absolutely necessary to communicate. Some of the other stutterers in the group subsequently reported that in their informal gatherings he was much more at ease but still showed signs of the behavior seen in the clinic.

In his speech he tolerated no stuttering whatever. He permitted no word to be spoken unless spoken fluently. That his speech was replete with phonation unrelated to the word being attempted was of little consequence as long as the word itself was unsullied by stuttering. One of the results of this was that Arthur maintained a constant stream of unproductive sound that served only to focus the attention of the listener and catch him up in the possibility that something was about to be said. It was this behavior that resulted in the feeling of never-endingness. For example, Arthur could produce a staccato schwa for a full three minutes before allowing himself to say the word "chair." Other instrumental behaviors even more remote to the speech act included eye-closing, a dropping of the chin to the right shoulder (much like the flinch in the face of a threatened blow) and a kind of swallowing sound made with the mouth closed. This latter sound was also capable of rapid production and was frequently prodromal to the staccato schwa, particularly at times of unusual communicative stress.

In his participation in the group, Arthur quickly established himself as low man. It was more difficult for him to carry out the assignments than anyone else. Yet the few times he did he showed marked improvement which served to goad the others on. Success did not goad Arthur, however, except to make him feel angry at the therapist because a successfully completed assignment meant that the therapist had probably been manipulating him, thus, depriving him of the chance to do it on his own. (As has been previously suggested, Arthur's therapy group paralled that of Alex. The therapy employed was essentially the same with a focus on successive approximations carried out by a series of written assignments leading to the giving up of avoidance, reduction of fear, modification of behavior and preparation for fluency.)

Before several months had passed, Arthur found himself completely outclassed by the other group members. He was still working unsuccessfully and arbitrarily to accomplish assignments that had been simple for the others. When new material was presented, Arthur was thus unable to profit from it. His attendance became sporadic and when he was at the group meetings the other members felt uneasy and somewhat guilty about their own feelings of success.

Finally, just before Thanksgiving, Arthur's student clinician made a special appointment with me to discuss him. She said that he was seriously thinking of giving up the therapy completely and had broken down with her and cried, upset over his lack of progress. The student's concern was one of personal puzzlement. She had never seen anyone like this before and wondered if everything was going to be all-right. She was basically a sympathetic person and was genuinely concerned about Arthur. She also indicated that her own role in his stuttering was unknown to her and that he found it very difficult to talk with her about it. This information was consistent with previous observations that Arthur did not talk easily about himself with others but made every effort to avoid sharing his feelings and reactions.

By the end of the appointment it was apparent to both the student clinician and myself that for Arthur to continue in therapy would not be profitable and that some other alternative to the present therapy plan would have to be worked out.

I consulted a colleague and explored the case at length. The following factors were considered: (1) Arthur's intense desire for complete independence despite his lack of ability to generate any significant change on his own, (2) the negative quality of his feelings toward authority figures as determined by his punitive relationship with his father, (3) his general difficulty in relating easily and openly to others, (4) the practical problem of his inability to change within the framework of the therapy as it was presently constituted, and (5) his inability to tolerate any disruptions of fluency other than those that were a product of behaviors completely and totally unrelated to the speech attempt.

It was finally decided that the best course of action would be to set Arthur out on his own. He was told to stop coming to the group meetings and to make weekly oral reports to himself via tape-recordings about his thoughts, his stuttering, and his feelings. These oral self-reports were to be supplemented by periodic, written autobiographical statements. At such points that Arthur felt he would like to talk with me, I would be available for consultation. Clearly a holding action was settled on in the face of what appeared to be insurmountable resistance.

Arthur remained in the area of the clinic until the end of the year. He subsequently left for a trip to Mexico and wrote to say he was planning to get married that spring.

Where then was the failure? From Arthur's point of view to say that he was little changed as the result of his experience with therapy would be generous. At best, he had been forced to the realization that he had come to the end of the therapeutic road. There was nowhere else for him to go. He had not been able to accept the demands imposed on him by the therapy, nor, and this is the key to the failure, had the therapist been able to accept the demands imposed by Arthur.

This clinical failure is the best possible example of the fallacious assumption that only one therapy for stuttering exists and that the person who stutters need not be considered except in a most casual and unimportant way. With this assumption, it was easy to fall into a trap that led me to believe that Arthur didn't respond to the therapy because he was unwilling to do so and, therefore, wasn't really motivated to change. That the therapy or the therapist might have been actively preventing him from changing by supporting a neurotic belief system antithetical to change was never really considered until problems began to arise. By then, help for Arthur within the context of the clinic was impossible.

The reasons for this are many and some of them are very obvious. In a clinic setting that demands student training as well as service, an effort is made to provide a training experience that can be made systematic and, therefore, routine. This allows for consistency in training and the development of training patterns that inculcate therapy techniques calculated to help most of the people most of the time. The exceptional case is culled out so as to prevent confusion and minimize the already high anxiety levels of student clinicians. When Arthur was examined in the diagnostic clinic, although there were some negative prognostic signs, *e.g.* his discomfort with people, his inability to tolerate his stuttering and so on, these were disregarded. It was as if his "squareness" was ignored in the hope that he would ultimately "fit" the round hole.

A less obvious reason relates to my own feelings of anxiety. In working with stutterers I have come to feel that my therapy makes sense. That is, it is a therapy that works. It helps stutterers. In retrospect I have the uncomfortable knowledge that with Arthur what was at stake was my belief in myself as a therapist and my therapy. Arthur became what is commonly referred to as a "challenge." I failed to recognize that Arthur's challenge was not one of finding the right technical therapeutic variation to apply to his stuttering but rather in allowing myself to work therapeutically with his inability to accept what I was offering. Thus, therapy instead of progressing deteriorated into a battle of wits. I became convinced that if I only tried harder to get him to do the things he had not yet done that it would all work out well in the end. Arthur tried harder to help me understand he couldn't do it. In retrospect, he gave me many signs of this. From the beginning he was unable to perform his assignments. He was uncommunicative in the group. He became a social isolate. He would argue occasionally with some feeling against the value of a specific assignment. On at least one occasion, he confessed to the group his weakness and inability to perform. Most important, his disruption of the smooth progress of therapy made me feel angry with him for being a "bad" patient. However, all of these things I ignored in favor of maintaining the status quo, and I protected myself from my discomfort by rationalizing my feelings about him. It was with some relief then that I saw him go. And it was with greater relief that I shared the responsibility for his leaving with a colleague. To say it again: I failed to provide Arthur with what he needed by attempting to make him fit into a fixed, arbitrary therapeutic mold.

In analyzing Arthur's total reaction to the therapy, I have found the work of Giffin (1967) on interpersonal trust in the communication process has helped me to assess Arthur's behavior in a more systematic way. I've also found it helpful because it seems to shed some light on the nature of the relationhip between Arthur and myself.

In brief, Giffin has defined interpersonal trust as the ". . . reliance upon the communication behavior of another person in order to achieve a desired but uncertain objective in a risky situation." (p. 105). He then breaks down this concept of trust into six dimensions that describe the listener's perceptions of the speaker. For clarity, I have substituted "therapist" for "speaker" and "patient" for "listener" in the following discussion.

The first dimension is that of therapist expertness. In considering this area, I remembered that none of the patients in the group, Arthur included, had had any previous contact with me. They had all been screened in the diagnostic clinic by someone else, and I was one of several therapists who might have been assigned to the group. Thus, my expertness was an unknown quantity, and any expertise assigned to me by the patients was a function of the authority vested in me by the university which maintained a speech clinic on its campus. Thus, Arthur only knew that the clinic *offered* competent, expert help for stutterers. He did not know that the help would not be expert enough to meet his needs when he first applied for therapy. It took about three months for Arthur's belief in our expertise to wear off.

The second dimension, the reliability of the therapist as a source of information coupled with the third dimension, the intentions of the therapist toward the patient, proved particularly significant in my understanding of Arthur. The belief that whatever gains he made had to be done on his own was most important to him. He had learned through painful experience that male authority figures were notoriously unreliable and given to peculiar motivations in their interactions with him. Arthur always weighed any guidance from others very carefully on a scale that tended to favor his own resources as more reliable and more consistent with his own best interests. Some of the time this scepticism was conscious and overt. But much of the time it remained unconscious and was revealed only as a projection. It was obvious that the reliability and the intentions of the therapist although technically unimpeachable, were immaterial in the face of Arthur's previous experience.

The personal dynamism of the therapist, that is, the energy level of the therapist during the communication process, is the fourth dimension. Again, to the extent that high energy levels could be interpreted by Arthur as typical of punitive male authority figures, the therapist could certainly be viewed as a person from whom help would be difficult to obtain. I am not passive in my therapy but demanding, almost aggressive, with high expectations about performance.

The fifth dimension, the majority opinion of the other patients about the therapist, may have been the only factor that kept Arthur in therapy at all. In general, the response of the group was positive, and the patients were all making significant and sometimes dramatic changes. In all likelihood this fact made it extremely difficult, if not incongruous, for Arthur to leave precipitously as he might have done in another setting.

The sixth dimension, the personal attraction of the therapist for the patient, that is the likeableness, friendliness and so on that is demonstrated by the therapist in the course of his patient contacts, was not clearly understood by me at the time, but I'm sure that it too contributed in a positive way to Arthur remaining in the group. In addition, it proved to be a critical factor that, as will be seen, bore fruit some months later when Arthur called me at the university.

Fifteen months after Arthur left the group, he contacted me at my office. He was frantic. His financee had broken their engagement. I made an appointment to see him, but before we could get together he sent me a letter apologizing for disturbing me and suggesting that he would be able to work things out on his own.

Two weeks later he called again and insisted once more on seeing me. He appeared at my office completely shaken and desperate. He had been unable to sleep, was virtually mute, had recurring, delusional fantasies of someone wanting to kill him by blowing up his car, had been fired from his job and had fought with his parents about the broken engagement. He pleaded tearfully for a chance to work with me again and repeatedly assured me that I was the only person he could trust.

I began seeing him on an individual basis. Within several weeks his anxiety had diminished, and he had begun to work on the central issue of his relationship with his father. This therapeutic program, in contrast to the previous one, never focussed on Arthur's specific speech performance. He has been permitted to use the therapy on his own terms, defining for himself what he needed to do, whether it be in the area of his stuttering or in the area of his interpersonal relationships. Recently it has been possible to help him understand the connections between the two, and he is beginning now to explore both with the recognition that they are really one entity.

Within the context of my thinking about stuttering, Arthur falls into a second category of stutterers, those for whom stuttering is a symptom of an anxiety process related to unacceptable, potentially punishable thoughts and feelings arising out of the developing patterns of childhood. Arthur's father was the major source of his conflict. In order to accept his father, Arthur had to deny his own integrity as a human being. However, if he rejected his father, Arthur only isolated himself from the possibility of developing productive human relationships that would afford him the opportunity to become a mature, adult male. That Arthur was unable to see that all men were not like his father was not surprising, just saddening. However, that he is again searching is what is important now.

I am relieved that my earlier failure with him did not destroy him. I would also like to think that it was not a complete failure. At the very least, I did something that warranted his returning to give me a second chance.

reference

Griffin, K., The contribution of studies of source credibility to a theory of interpersonal trust in the communication process. *Psychological Bulletin,* 68, 104-120, 1967.

A CLINICAL SUCCESS: DON
CLINICIAN: C. VAN RIPER

introduction

In reviewing the case folders of some of the stutterers with whom I had worked successfully, it became immediately apparent that my clinical notes and impressions as recorded therein were far too sketchy and incomplete to provide an adequate picture of the actual dynamics of the therapy. Moreover, I did not entirely trust my memory. It is difficult enough to recognize the shifting needs, the transient urgencies, the momentary impacts, the misjudgments and failures, yes even the successful interactions which characterize the therapeutic relationship while it is taking place; to try to remember them after a lapse of time is almost impossible. One recalls the major problems encountered, the crucial experiences which apparently preceded a spurt of progress, and, if the clinical notes are fairly complete, the therapist at least knows what he did. But why he did what he did and what happened when he did it have gone with the snows of yesteryear. Accordingly, I decided to undertake the treatment of a stutterer especially for the purpose of the present project. I did not have much time, four months at the most, and at the best I would only work with the case a half hour a day, five days a week. Even this was opposed by my physician who felt that therapy involved too much stress on a heart that was having difficulty.

The selection of the stutterer with whom to work presented some ambivalence at first. I hesitated to work with one whose prognosis was too unfavorable, and there were several in the clinic who apparently would be good prospects. The matter was resolved, however, when one morning I met Don and heard him stuttering so severely I could scarcely bear it. I had begun to work with this young man as a member of a group a few months before my heart attacks. Don was one of the most severe stutterers I have ever known, and his progress in therapy had been minimal even when I was his group therapist. There in the clinic that morning he took twenty minutes to tell me he was worse than he had ever been and that he had only one more year before he graduated. After I had given up my clinical duties, others on our staff had worked with Don without any success or progress. He told me sadly that he had given up any hope of ever being able to talk without his paroxysms.

the stutterer

A brief synopsis of personal data on Don would run as follows: Age 21; onset of stuttering during third year of life; began gradually; parents could not account for onset in terms of any traumatic experience; had been speaking in short sentences by two years; no major illnesses or accidents; two older brothers, one older sister and two younger sisters, none of whom stuttered. There was no history of the disorder in the family; no major sibling conflicts. Father was pastor of a fairly large church in Arizona and made a comfortable living. His basic roles were those of provider and disciplinarian. To his family he seemed aloof. Don said, "My father did not ever seem close to us. Perhaps he had to be unfair to his children. My father is very intelligent, cultured, outwardly friendly and outgoing to his parishioners, but he could be very blunt; he said what he thought. Couldn't show much affection. My speech bothered him, but he wouldn't ever talk about it." The mother was warm and affectionate, devoted to the father and to the church; hard working. "She was always concerned about my stuttering, always tried to help. Saw to it I got speech therapy and reminded me of what I had to do. She carried out any suggestions made to her by therapists. She liked me but worried about me. A very fine person."

Don did well in school. Intelligent. College grades were A's and B's despite his inability to communicate. In high school Don took an active part in scouting and athletics and was successful. Had summer jobs and earned enough money to take care of most of his personal needs. He was a member of a closely knit group of boys during high school and had some satisfying group experiences. Members of the group did not penalize his stuttering and accepted him despite it. Had one close chum. Little dating in high school. "Couldn't ask the girls out because of my speech, but I've made up for it here in college. I get plenty of turndowns, but I go out enough." Don achieved a fairly close relationship with one college girl, a major in speech correction. "I managed to pin her, but I think it will break up. Sometimes I lose interest and so does she."

Don is a major in accounting in business school and for the past year has served as the paid business manager of the university yearbook. "I didn't get it because of my speech but because the books were in a mess, and they needed somebody to straighten them out. I've stuttered like hell, but it's been good for me; kept me from withdrawing from people; made me use the phone."

Don says that he has been in therapy ever since he was in kindergarten. "All that ever happened was that I steadily grew worse." Most of this therapy was administered by public school therapists in groups with articulation cases. Also worked with student majors in a college training center and for one semester with one of the professors. "They had me intone and relax; no good." Had a few interviews with a psychiatrist during high school who suggested that he should have more psychiatric help when he went to college. The stuttering has remained consistently severe since early in high school.

On clinic entrance, Don was administered the MMPI, the TAT and the Bender Gestalt. On the MMPI, he performed within normal limits except for a slight deviation on the Si (Social introversion) scale. The TAT revealed no major findings except some unsatisfied sexual fantasies. On the Bender Gestalt, perseveration and response rigidity were prominent. Exploratory interviews in some depth gave no indication of psychopathology. The Sheehan modification of Rotter's Incomplete Sentence Test and several other tests indicated low aspiration levels. On the W-A-Y test, his major roles were: "A stutterer"; "Don Z."; and "A Man." Tests of motor coordination gave normal performance except for the presence of frequent fine tremors especially in bimanual activities.

The symptomatic picture presented was as follows: Don stuttered on over fifty percent of his words in oral reading and the percentage was much higher in propositional speech even in a relatively non-stressful situation. He showed very little adaptation on rereadings or on repeating individual words, often an increase. There was no reduction in frequency under low frequency masking at 80 dB though there was some decrease in the duration of his blockings. The average duration of his moments of stuttering in oral reading was 4 seconds; the longest one was 28. In propositional speech the durations were longer. Occasionally he would just have to quit speaking.

Except for the use of "um but" or "oh" or "um" or "ah" which he used to get started, there were few avoidances. "I see no point in substituting an easier word like the other guys often do. I don't have any. If I try one, I get hung up on that too." As with most of the very severe stutterers, he had few specific phonemic or word fears, but his situation fears were very intense, often to the point of panic. Usually, Don plunged directly into the utterance, went into a prolonged tremor of the articulators, squeezed shut his eyes, jerked his jaw open very widely to interrupt the tremor, then did it again and again. Great tension accompanied this behavior and often it overflowed to the limbs and trunk. In his paroxynsms, he would even stagger. Most of the grostesque behavior apparently seemed to serve as interruptor and escape devices. The tremors of the lips and jaws, which we were able to record electromyographically, ranged in frequency from 7 to 18 per second, with most of them oscillating at the first value. Often as a result of his longer blockings, he would become completely exhausted. Airflow was often interrupted at the laryngeal level as well as by the occluded tongue or lips. In some of his worst moments of stuttering, the tongue would protrude violently and show marked tremor.

Despite the severity of his overt stuttering behavior and the many unpleasant responses it had evoked from listeners, Don's attitudes toward his problem were unusually non-morbid. On the Ammons'-Johnson Attitude Scale, his responses were those of a very mild stutterer. He was quite objective and accepting and even analytical when he listened to his audiorecordings of his severe stuttering. He attributed this to all the therapy he had had but when he saw himself on videotape, he was shocked. "I never knew how bad I was," he said. We have observed much of the same lack of affect in other very severe stutterers. Like them, Don had built a sort of insulation and denial and disregard as a buffer against the self confrontation and the confrontation of others. "For one thing, when I have my eyes shut, I can't see how other people are reacting to this monster," he said and laughed a bit grimly. As the tests had shown, his aspiration levels were low with regard to therapy. "I don't have much hope any more. Too many people have worked me over. I'll try, but I'm not expecting much from you or myself. If I can ever talk easily, I'll be surprised. But I'll get along anyway. I've learned to live with it."

the therapy

When I asked the therapist's old question: "What does he need now?" it was obvious that somehow I must try to find and mobilize the latent motivation which exists in even the sorriest stutterer. The prospect was not favorable. Frustrating as the stuttering was, he had, as he said, learned to bear it. In his previous experience with me in group therapy, he had shown little initiative; he had often failed to do the assignments given to the group or had fulfilled them with token efforts at best. He had little faith in any therapist and small hope. The facts that he was nearing the end of his college career and would probably never again have another opportunity to have therapy and that he had seen other stutterers with whom I had worked successfully were about the only positive influences on which I could count. All of his acquaintances expected him to stutter and so did he. Stuttering was deeply buried both in his language and in his living activities. Nevertheless, I was certain that if I could create a favorable therapeutic situation, I could help him. This faith I have always had as a clinician, and it stems from my own personal experience. I still remember vividly what a severe stutterer and how tangled emotionally I once was. When I see any stutterer, I remember my own unfavorable prognosis, my own weakness, my lack of hope, and when I do, I find in the case before me strengths and potentials which I did not have. If I could do what I have done, then surely this person could do as much. This is very real faith, and I suspect it has played a large part in any success I have had as a clinician. In my first interview with Don, I expressed all of his doubts even better than he could have done, but I also made sure that he felt the impact of my certainty that he had within him the potential for healing himself. I painted no rosy picture of what had to be done; I painted it black. He would have to make an extreme effort and there would be moments of weakness and despair. We would have to contrive to put as many odds as we could muster in his favor. I would be his guide out of the swamp of communicative frustration, but I could not carry him. I let him know that my physicians had insisted that I do no therapy but was accepting him as a case anyway. I told him I could only give him half an hour a day and that if I had too much angina, I would have to abandon the work, but I wanted to try anyway.

At this time, May 1967, Don was living with a roommate in an apartment. He had finished the spring semester at the university and had a job in a factory from three in the afternoon until midnight so that he could earn enough to go back to school in the fall. To create a more favorable situation, I suggested that he move out to my farm where my son's apartment in the garage was vacant. He had an old sports car so transportation was not a problem and that way he could save money. I would give him the use of the apartment and breakfast, and I would hold a daily conference with him in my study at eight o'clock each morning. In addition, he would spend an hour each morning with Lucy, a graduate student whom I had been grooming for a supervisory position in a university and with whom I was working closely. Their sessions would be audio or video taped so I could review their interaction. Occasionally I would ask Don to appear before my class in Stuttering. I made it clear that he would have to spend most of his free time working on his speech. This was the plan I presented. Don accepted it with some reluctance, I felt. He did not desire to live alone; the prospect of the obligation and commitment did not appear attractive. But he moved out and we began.

first two weeks

I felt it vital to begin with intensive therapy, with a schedule of activities which would require almost all his free time apart from working in the factory or sleeping. Token efforts such as he had shown in the past would give us no chance for success. There was need to create as total an involvement in therapy as we could achieve. Accordingly in our first session I presented him with the following daily therapy plan, explained the rationale behind each activity, and had him do a sample of each in my presence. I asked him to explain and demonstrate each before Lucy, the graduate student clinician, and told him that on Friday he was to appear before my stuttering class and do the same thing. I pointed out that

I had set no quotas or amounts for any single activity but that, if he wished to have the morning conference with me, he had to have done something on each one. I suggested that he keep a log of all achievement, or failures to perform, and also that he be able to report his feelings about the experiences, about himself, and about me.

therapy plan first two weeks

I. To establish models and nuclei of fluent speech:
   a. Echo speech in pantomime while listening to other speakers.
   b. Oral reading of conversational speech (plays, interviews, etc.)
   c. Free association aloud to self.
   d. Completing unfinished sentences from cards.
   e. Paraphrase from reading loud to self.
   f. Speaking impromptu from topic cards.
II. Tremor control with Lucy and me.
   a. Voluntary stuttering on syllables so that deceleration of tremors occurs.
   b. Slow motion utterance of words phonemically.
   c. Progressive relaxation of tensed mouth postures and revising them until correct posture is attained.
   d. Negative practice on surges of tension with utterance coming only when relaxation has been accomplished.
III. Eliminating the reinforcement of stuttering behaviors:
   a. Refusing to continue communication after blocking until you have counted slowly to ten and then had an equivalent period of non-counting silence. Just wait. Tolerate frustration.
   b. Collect instances in which you first integrate the fractured sound, then attempt and integrate the syllable, then the word, then the phrase and finally the sentence. If failure at any point occurs, go back to the beginning of the sequence until finally the whole sentence is spoken without any loss of control whatsoever.
   c. To reduce the reinforcement which comes from repression and detachment, make prewritten phone calls which can be used over and over again: "This is Don Z. May I speak to Nancy?" Do these before a mirror and while tape recording. Continue these for a set period of time but stop as soon as success occurs, even if the period is not up.
   d. Replay all recorded phone calls while first alone and then with someone else, saying the stuttered words correctly while speaking in unison with yourself.
IV. While eating:
   a. Say a feared word without stuttering before taking a bite of anything; then a phrase once you have succeeded, then a sentence. In this work first by mouthing it in pantomime, then whispering, then saying aloud.
   b. While working with Lucy, at the first recognition of fear, shut your eyes, and put your fingers in your ears, as you rehearse your attempt at normal utterance. Do not open them until you are fairly sure you can say them without struggle. You must learn to revise your abnormal preparatory sets.
V. Learn to beat the delayed feedback machine and work on it every weekday.

My clinical notes on the first two weeks of therapy may be summarized in this way. After some initial testing to see if I really meant what I had said about doing all of the activities, and after missing a few conferences, Don began to do a good job. By the end of the first week, he was able to talk fluently to himself without stuttering, something that had not previously occurred. He would get up early, walk out in the fields reading orally and paraphrasing, shouting, doing free association, paraphrasing, making speeches from the topic cards. I had provided his apartment with a telephone and a big tape recorder, and he did his shadowing or echo speech of utterances (usually the commercials from his radio) which he had previously recorded. The unfinished sentences were ones which I had provided, most of which were coded so as to evoke some self confrontation or to express his emotions. His verbalized thinking improved markedly under this regime but most important of all, he found pleasure in this strong fluency. He had never known it before. With all his doubts about transfer, the new models of good speech even in self talk had their impact.

The assigned activities in tremor control presented more difficulty. They were performed both while alone and with Lucy at first and by the end of the second week in telephoning strangers. He found it very distasteful to attempt to throw himself into one of his jaw, tongue or lip tremors since even when alone they tended to become involuntary and perseverative. Of all his stuttering behaviors, this to him seemed the core of his difficulty. In our conferences, we worked out desensitization schedules which eventuated in cumulative successes. This too was highly motivating. By the end of the second week, he was reporting times when he had been able to do the various tremor controls even at work and in speaking to strangers though there were still more failures than successes. He found, while telephoning in his apartment, that by using a mirror he could modify the tremors more easily when watching himself. Their durations decreased. He confessed a tiny ray of hope.

The third group of activities presented the most difficulty and although he tried, Don was completely unable to follow a moment of stuttering with the prescribed silence except occasionally with me or Lucy and never in any other situation. Time pressure was evidently one of his major problems, as it is with most stutterers, but during these first two weeks, Don seemed completely unable to cope with it. Lucy and I verbalized for him his distress and accepted the failures permissively, but it was evident that we would have to approach this problem more gradually. The other activities in this group showed increasing improvement. Occasionally Don was able to integrate his fractured speech when he did not think he could. He reported instances of surprise when expected stuttering did not occur or when it was shorter or milder than he had anticipated.

In the morning, Don was always starved. He would fix himself a good breakfast and then bring it into my study. I would then set up a bit of behavior to be rewarded by one small bite of egg or toast or one sip of coffee or orange juice. Often the food got cold before it was eaten and sometimes the conference period ended with much of it untouched. As he gradually became more successful, however, we set up small quotas which had to be achieved before he took food. By this approximation to operant therapy (or a therapeutic infantile feeding situation, etc.), we attacked his eye closings, jaw jerks, abnormal mouth postures, tongue protrusions, the "um-but" starters and many other of the instrumental responses which formed so large a part of his abnormality. Significantly, we did not apply it to the tremors themselves. Occasionally, I would eat my breakfast with Don, and he could deprive me of a bite or sip by being able to say a word, phrase, or sentence without any of these reactions even though stuttering occurred. He enjoyed those sessions.

By the end of the second week, he was becoming comparatively fluent with me. There were still many moments of stuttering, but they were shorter and usually without too much tension or overflow. Some very visible improvement was shown also with Lucy and when he spoke to my class in stuttering. Also, by the end of the second week, he was able to speak completely fluently under delayed auditory feedback, thanks to a desensitization schedule in which we gradually increased the delay time and intensity from values which had no effect to the critical .18 seconds and 80 dB where disruption was most apparent. In this training, as soon as we saw signs of breakdown or rhythmic changes, we went back to the basal fluency level. Often to get it we would have to speak in unison with him.

third and fourth weeks

A new regime was begun at the beginning of the third week of therapy. By this time, Don was working well. He was also highly motivated and the comparative fluency which he now experienced with Lucy and me was, as he said, "sweet in the mouth." Though he still had many severe stutterings away from the farm or speech clinic with which he could not cope at all, I felt he was ready for another push. He had frequently expressed the fear that the improvement was too localized and that he didn't seem to be able to do much on his own, that he "went haywire" into the old spasmodic behaviors when stress situations occurred at work or play. "The sword hangs over my head and you hold the shield." I felt he was asking for more opportunities to work on his speech in outside situations and for less dependency. One always respects these silent cries and while I felt that some "flight into health" dynamics were occurring, I designed the following therapy plan to give him more responsibility and more contact with the outside world.

1. When the alarm clock rings, lie there in bed and review the preceding day's performance in terms of the basic aims of the therapy. Ask yourself "What do I need to do to make more progress? Where am I falling short and what can I do to change?" Then dress, go over to the tape recorder and dictate your summary of this thinking and your plans for the day expressed in terms of maximum and minimum achievement goals. Bring this to our conference. I want to hear it.

2. Listen to some of your old tapes which have severe stuttering on them. Amplify them loudly, turning up the volume control every time you hear some stuttering.

3. Prepare twenty cards with topics on them which have special emotional significance for you. (Examples: "The Future," "Guilt," etc.). Go out into the barn and orate to the cats on the topic of a card pulled out at random, trying to keep going for at least five minutes and using the same kind of speech you employ in beating the delayed feedback machine.

4. In our conference, we will first play the tape and talk about it, then you will report to me the successes and failures of the preceding day which you will have jotted down on cards carried by you constantly. We will use the same sort of operant conditioning program as before, but from now on you will get your bite or sip only after you have been able to say whole sentences. The hierarchy will be to say them in pantomime, in a whisper, and then aloud.

5. After the conference, return to the apartment and make phone calls asking for information, prewriting the first sentences thereof and underlining all words stuttered upon. After the phone calls have been completed, tape record all sentences on which stuttering occurred, repeating each until they are spoken fluently at least five times. Then say each one again twice, first while duplicating your former stuttering and secondly while saying it fluently. If you have failures in this, redo them till you have success.

6. At the clinic, first practice shadowing or echo speech with Lucy, then work out on the delayed feedback apparatus, then, with her observing, start the basic assignment for the day: thirty phone calls to strangers with five deducted from the quota for each success. Success is here defined as stuttering without facial grimaces, eye closings or jaw jerks. Tremors alone should not be considered as failures unless you stop and start them over. Move forward.

7. Using a mirror, and placing your chin on your hand with your elbow on the table, work for proprioceptive monitoring, beginning slowly, then going faster but always feeling your mouth. Do some of this with your eyes closed; some with eyes closed and fingers in ears.

8. Negative practice on short sudden jaw jerks on the first words to five strangers. After you have done so, stop, then say the whole sentence over again the way you should.

9. Practice tremoring of the jaw, the lips, and the tongue, first in silence, then on an appropriate word. Be sure to hold the posture steady before stopping and saying the word, and hold it for some time. Check in mirror to make sure.

10. Three pages of careful and strongly monitored simultaneous talking and writing. Think out the sentence before beginning to write. If confusion comes, don't count it, but begin again. Encircle all words on which any stuttering occurs and write them out.

In addition to the above program, I also enlisted Virginia (Jinny), Don's girl friend, in the therapy by asking her to reward Don for behaviors which indicated progress by smiles or affectionate touches. Since she was a major in speech therapy and knew what

Don's assignments were, and he usually drove her around in his car each day, I felt that this sort of positive reinforcement might have some effect. Anyway, Don felt that it did. Each night after work at midnight he would phone her. Once I overheard him doing so. He was watching himself in the mirror and working hard on his speech. How Jinny was reinforcing him then I don't know.

In reviewing my clinical notes, it is quite apparent that during this period Don made another real bit of progress. His general fluency increased not only with me and Lucy but also with my wife who had usually evoked severe stuttering when they spoke alone together. For the first time she noted a definite improvement. Telephoning had always been an especially difficult situation for Don. Many of his listeners had hung up on him and some strangers had been very impatient and even insulting. By using this feared situation we were able to bring the outside world into the therapy room and apartment and since he had to formulate the messages and make the contacts without my being present, he had to accept more responsibility. Moreover, by making a decrease in the quota of thirty phone calls contingent upon success (as defined) we mobilized the forces of negative reinforcement. During the first week of this schedule, Don seldom was able to decrease the quota by more than five or ten calls despite strenuous efforts to prepare himself for the pre-written utterance. Each morning he said he woke up dreading this assignment and hating me and hoping for the weekend when he could tell me and speech therapy to go to hell. I grinned and ate a piece of toast.

The second day of the second week, he reported having only to make ten phone calls because he had had four successes on his first phone calls. He was lying and we both knew it although I said nothing. I arranged to have Lucy take him downtown that morning and to call me at my office. His stuttering was severe and completely uncontrolled, as bad as it had ever been, so I said, quietly and calmly, "Sorry, Don, but I won't listen to speech like that. I know what you can do." And I hung up the receiver. Lucy reported later that Don reacted as though he had been "hit in the face." But after about half an hour he called me again and, working very hard, he spoke very well. This was apparently a crucial experience. Our conference the following morning involved more psychotherapy than speech therapy. We omitted the "operant conditioning" but had some counterconditioning at work because I had fixed a huge breakfast which he wolfed as he got a lot of hate and guilt and doubt out of him and into my accepting receptacle. From this time onward, his performance on the telephone improved remarkably. That Friday I had him make a phone call to the airport about a reservation for me before my entire stuttering class and he did well. This was a large trophy since the week before in a similar situation he had failed abjectly.

During this period, Don also made great progress in proprioceptive monitoring of his fluent speech. He was feeling it rather than listening for the gaps and abnormality of his stuttering. The fluent speech had stimulus value now. The rate of his speech slowed down; it was more conscious, deliberate, stronger. The gross secondary struggle behaviors had disappeared though often they still existed in miniature. He talked more. At times he overexaggerated the articulation in the same manner that he used in beating the delayed auditory feedback, and I cautioned him to speak more naturally while still attending to proprioception.

The tremors were still evident though usually unaccompanied by overflow or interrupter reactions, but they were shorter. About this time, Don began to develop phonemic fears, a sign which I felt indicated progress, and also some easy automatic repetitions of syllables similar to those which mark the initial stages of the disorder. Often these occurred without awareness, and I did not bring them to his attention. A quotation from one of his tape recordings at the end of the first month of therapy will illustrate his primary concerns. "The main things that bug me now are the way that my tremors keep running. I don't know how to stop them or control them without just quitting entirely and starting again and then they come back. They run away with me. Another thing is on my vowel sound or H-words. I open my mouth and it starts vibrating but nothing comes out. No sound and sometimes not even breath. I'm stuck down in my throat. Sometimes I can get some breath out, but it shuts off suddenly before the sound comes. I need help on this. I also need help in shifting from one sound to another smoothly. Always want to jerk. And I still have times, like down at the Brown and Gold office, when someone makes a demand on me for speech suddenlike. Too many times I forget everything I've learned and just go into my old crazy stuff."

second month

As we reviewed the clinical situation together at the beginning of this period it became apparent that Don should start being his own therapist. He had begun to invent assignments for himself in addition to those I had given him. He had gained the ability to evaluate his performance fairly realistically and with insight. In our conferences he had asked to leave the operant scheduling so that he could more freely discuss the problems he had encountered and his performances. He had cut down his working hours so he could have more time to work on his speech and with Lucy he was taking complete charge of all the sessions, using her primarily as an observer and discussant. In his sessions before my class he was now playing the role of instructor and information giver not only when I absented myself for a short period of time but also when I was present. He was able to consider and reject the suggestions I made which to him seemed inappropriate. His relationship with his girl had also changed, she told me. He was becoming more independent and aggressive. He was ogling other girls. All of these bits of information and many more indicated a need for change.

Our next conferences were spent in an intensive review of what had happened and the problems which remained. I redefined my role as being a consultant and his as being his own therapist. He was to devise his own subgoals and quotas again in terms of maximum and minimum achievement. He was to formulate them in writing prior to our morning conference and to provide a written report of the previous day's experiences. I purchased a high fidelity portable tape recorder for his use, and he was to record all of his speech during the day and listen to it before he went to bed. His first day's report is as follows:

Things went quite well today. I got my program half-way organized and my speech was fairly good. I had a lot of fluent speech, but after listening to the conversations I recorded, I didn't have as much voluntaries as I should have. I also found that I did not keep too accurate records.

The program I have laid out will need a little revising. It still is not entirely comprehensive enough because I haven't put all the things in that I need to do.

The day began over at the bookstore where I had some problems. After listening to the playback of this conversation, I think part of the problem was my attempts weren't strong enough. This problem appeared several other times during the day, especially during my good times. If I speak too weakly, I tremor.

Besides the bookstore, I went to the Union, did BROWN & GOLD business which included about five incoming and five outgoing calls and several situations in the administration building; Miller's; and Sears. Of course, there was also conversation at work.

The main problems that arose were I didn't work on all phases of my program (I was a bit unorganized) and my speech was weak and rushed at times. Of course, I had a lot of tremors, but they are expected, and I did work on all most all of them.

I felt real good after the day was over. I felt that I made quite a bit of progress and that I am off my plateau and moving. I was surprised when I listened to the playback of the conversations which I recorded because I had more involuntary speech and "um-buts" than I realized.

Today I am going to concentrate on keeping better records, on the strong voluntary speech, and different ways of resisting the time pressure.

Nevertheless, as I had anticipated, the change had its repercussions. That weekend Don found the going tougher as his report indicates:

This weekend all hell broke loose, and I managed to take some giant steps backwards. The main thing that happened was that I became too impatient and did not demand proper speech, so the bad speech got an unhealthy dose of reinforcement.

The one thing that could really characterize my speech this weekend was tremors I couldn't get hold of. They would even be present when I pantomimed. After making several half-hearted attempts, I would use one of my old tactics to get out of the tremor, gaping or jerking, eyes shut. I really didn't do much actual therapy work this weekend. I felt kind of lazy, and I think this was one reason I had such a bad time.

Another thing I noticed was my speech, especially when it was tremoring, sounded very light, like I was really nervous about something. The thing that bothers me is that I can't locate any major problem area that I think has me especially worried, except maybe my progress with my speech.

Today I am going to revert to the basics—self-talk; oral reading; simultaneous writing and talking; holding of tremors; pantomime; the syllable and saying that, then the word, and voluntary speech.

The month was a fairly stormy one for Don. Periods of progress were succeeded by marked regression, but the oscillations each time resulted in higher levels of performance. For a few days after his car broke down, he lapsed into a deep depression and apathy and did little, missing several conferences for I steadfastly refused to see him unless he had prepared the daily therapy plans, reports and had recorded all of his utterance. These instances were rare, however. Most of our sessions consisted of a discussion of the playback of tapes, or the plans and reports. I verbalized his feelings when he could not do so and reflected them when he did. At times I offered the reassurance of my faith in his potential to work out of his difficulties. I never suggested an assignment during this period, but I provided information and helped him analyze his behavior and attitudes. A fairly typical exchange is illustrated by the following excerpt from a session I recorded in my study. We were replaying his tape of the preceding day's speech.

Don: Hear that? That's what I'm doing too often. A vowel word. I'm silent but my mouth is ajar and my jaw is jumping. Nothing coming out, no air. How do I get air coming or sound?

Van Riper: Yup, these are the tough ones. You're trying to pour water out of a corked bottle, and you're pressing down on the cork. Where's the cork?

Don: Down here (pointing to his larynx).

Van Riper: But the word finally did come out, didn't it? You finally got the air and sound coming. How did you do it then?

Don: Let me hear it again. (Reverses and replays that portion of the tape.) Oh, yeah. There's that buzz just before the sound comes. You told me about that once. What do you call it?

Van Riper: The vocal fry.

Don: Yeah, vocal fry, like this. (Demonstrates) You mean I should do it on purpose when I'm blocked so I can ease out?

Van Riper: Why don't you explore that kind of a release today when you have some of that kind of stuttering and see what happens. There are some other things too about what happens as you come out of those silent tremors which you could profit from knowing.

Don: And you aren't going to tell me?

Van Riper: Nope.

During the first week of this month we videotaped several of the clinical sessions Don had with Lucy, let him see them, and analyzed the behavior. As we had found before, the use of videotape playback has a profound effect upon stutterers, creating an objectivity that cannot be achieved in any other way. Mirror observation has some of this utility, but the same segment of behavior cannot be repeated over and over again. We asked Don to shadow his own image and speech but to try to stutter fluently whenever he saw his old abnormality. He soon came to do this very well and developed insights into the inappropriateness of his struggle behavior very rapidly. He became fascinated by his tremors, studying them. In his videotaping sessions with Lucy he became very careful and remarkably fluent. We asked him why? "Maybe it's pride or maybe I just can't bear looking like such a fool with my mouth jumping up there on the monitor. I've got to fight like the devil to keep the jerks and tremors out, but I'm finding that I can. I don't just have to let it go crazy."

After four of these sessions, I asked Don to go over to the studio and to summarize this therapy to date on videotape—and without Lucy or me being present. He was to speak on this tape for a period of at least half an hour. Don reported great fear of the situation, but it turned out to be another one of those crucial experiences, the turning points in therapy, which all clinicians hope for. I noticed immediately afterward a marked gain in fluency and when I viewed the videotape I understood. The first word that Don spoke was a very long grotesque moment of stuttering. It seemed to last interminably, and I could see the dismay, fear and shock flooding over him. He tried and tried to release himself, resorting to all his old monster behaviors until finally he uttered the word. He was obviously very shaken but then deliberately went back to that word, got into another tremor, and slowly and carefully smoothed it out and spoke it strongly. Then he did it again, this time without tremor or abnormality but carefully. And then he spoke with complete fluency for the rest of the half hour of taping. He has never forgotten that experience; he says it changed his life. He saw a new self.

About the middle of the month we terminated Don's sessions with Lucy without difficulty. As he said, "She's learning more from me than I am from her. I can do my own observing now and these damned tapes keep me honest." At this time, I asked my wife, who is an excellent and experienced speech therapist with stutterers, to query Don occasionally about what was happening in some of the stuttering he was having in speaking with her. She was to make no suggestions, merely to aid in the confrontation and exploration of his behavior. We also began to have him occasionally take supper with us and our guests so that we could observe him in these situations.

By the end of the month, Don had achieved an average fluency in most of his situations which was far better than he had ever known, and he was thoroughly enjoying it. In stress situations, some of his old severe stutterings occasionally occurred, but he was talking copiously. He was also speaking very fast and, at times, almost in a cluttering fashion. There were many short little facsimilies of his old behavior, tiny jerks, eye closures, flicks of the tongue, tremors. Only occasionally would he employ the proprioceptive monitoring of his normal speech. The "um-buts" increased. I knew from the signs that trouble was brewing. Usually in such a situation I would have permitted the relapse to occur so that he could recognize his folly and learn from it, but because our time was growing short, I decided otherwise.

Accordingly, I took a day off and spent most of the morning with him. I confronted Don with the picture of what I had been seeing and told him that unless a drastic about face took place immediately, I was terminating the therapy and he could move back to town. I played several of the tapes, pointing out exactly what I meant, and I told him that I would, thenceforth, listen to the tape of the previous day's speech before deciding whether we would have a conference or not, that when he talked to me he would have to talk carefully and use what he had learned or I would refuse to listen to him. I instructed my wife to follow the same policy.

After the first shock, Don accepted my comments surprisingly well, almost with relief. He told me that I was an old bastard, but he knew that what I was saying was right. Nevertheless, he did not come in for a conference for two days. His verbatim report is as follows:

In certain respects I am quite disappointed with my performance these last three days. Before starting to prepare this report, I was relatively satisfied with what I had done. I felt like I had done more this weekend than any previous weekend. I had a good solid session of work on Friday, and I managed to keep up effort at work that evening. On Saturday I actively sought out situations and did many different things with my speech. I thought that the therapist-self was starting to overpower the stutterer-self.

When I started to prepare this report, I tried to find the card I kept tally with on Friday. I couldn't find it, so I had to prepare my graph by estimating. I also listened to the playback of the things I recorded on Friday and was very disappointed. A lot of my speech was just "yak" speech. The disappointing thing is that I tried to concentrate on the voluntariness of the speech.

I also counted four "um-buts" on the tape.

The positive thing that showed up was a lot of integration and motor imagery. I also did work on resisting the time pressure during the actual conversation.

On Saturday, I feel that I did more actual therapy-type work than any previous Saturday. I was still working on the time pressure on the voluntary speech and on integration as a means of controlling the tremor. It went quite well and when I talked to John Adams that afternoon I was able to show him a lot of improvement over last Saturday's speech. The integration was coming. I don't think I was too susceptible to time pressure, and my speech was more voluntary although it was still too fast. I won't even try to estimate my work on Saturday. Sunday, I didn't do as much although I had one speaking experience with a fraternity brother in which I had some old type movements and contortions.

I feel that my therapy plans do need some major revisions. The first thing I am going to do is cut out the self-talking I have included. I want to replace this with a five to ten minute warm up period which will be done at the beginning of each day. I also feel the need to work on these tremors a lot more. I need both to reduce the fear and to learn to release them easily. John Adams told me that he did a lot of a tremor-smooth-tremor-smooth routine. I feel this would be a great help to me. I am also going to have to insert some negative practice on my "um-buts."

I feel that I have made some definite, concrete progress, although I am letting a lot of good situations and bad speech get by. Thanks, Dr. Van.

Don worked hard and intelligently for the next three weeks, concentrating on one problem after another. My role increasingly became that of a listener as he explained what he had done and why. He was in active charge of his own therapy. I stopped listening to his recordings but we went over his daily reports together in our conferences. Only rarely did I offer any suggestions. Usually, I just drew him out, had him amplify, helped him think more deeply by my questions. Two of his reports reflect this period fairly clearly:

Today was a very interesting day. I attempted to fake tremors so I could learn how to control them and ended up having less control than before. What I felt was interesting was that many of the old mannerisms, escape attempts, lip closures, and sudden jaw movements were apparent. Instead of helping overcome these tendencies, I had a double dose of them.

I am rather glad this thing happened today because it gave me a lot of insight into what happens to set off the tremors. I think I was finally learning how to overcome the tremor by relaxation and integration.

The two things which really set off the tremors were the "tremor-smooth-tremor-smooth" turn on and turn off sequence and the easy stuttering. Many times these would go off into the real thing. It is interesting to note that I did not complete my quota for integrated words. I know I need to have a real strong dose of the integration. What I want to do tomorrow is to follow every tremor-smooth, etc., sequence with a highly voluntary and integrating production of the same word. I will also try that on the sentence right after I have a sentence of easy stuttering. I'm coming, Dr. Van.

Today went a lot better than yesterday. The big difference was in the control of the tremor. I had both real and faked. I followed the blocking tremoring by purposeful integration, many times pantomiming before integrating. I got a clear feeling of what is the wrong way, and this is the right way.

I enjoyed my voluntary stuttering. This was both an imitation of my old and different varieties of stuttering. I would try this on both single words and whole conversations. In the next situation I would try to be sure I had strong integration to compare.

After my warm-up reading, I made some phone calls like to the vocational rehabilitation office, a doctor's office, a secretary over on campus, as well as several others. These calls provided a good springboard for the rest of the day. I then did some work over at the university, mostly in the Union. In the afternoon I spent over an hour at Westwood Shopping Center.

I enjoyed today's work because I showed a lot of progress over yesterday. I have given myself a large dose of work on the heart of my problem (tremors), and I was able to stand up and fight it.

Tomorrow I am going to plan on doing basically the same things. I am also going to use a lot of bouncing at different rates. This should help to build up my control since if they go fast they often get out of control and I have tremors. I am also going to have to work from the other end of the problem as well. In order to do this, I will vary each conversation— *i.e.*, in the first conversation, I will be concentrating on gaining control of the tremor, and on the second conversation I will strive for complete sentences with a high degree of voluntariness.

Toward the end of the month, Don was speaking so well that he was receiving a good many compliments from people who had known him formerly. One of these who was impressed with his growth was a girl who had come to us from Hong Kong to overcome her stuttering problem and to prepare herself as a speech therapist. Don saw her frequently and often she accompanied him on some of his self-therapy situations. With the encouragement of her therapist, Don helped her a little, and it strengthened his newly found role. He began to ask me questions involving clinical judgment and probabilities. He again began to graph his work output and compute his success failure ratios. He studied some learning theory and surprised me by applying it to his own problems. His father and mother visited him one weekend in my absence and a letter from them reported their pleasure in hearing Don speaking well for the first time. Don said it was a bit hard at first to talk to his father but that he had done well.

It was during this period that Don began to concentrate on modifying, releasing and preventing his tremors and on resisting time pressure. Much of his situation fear had subsided. Even in talking to his foreman in the factory he was able to speak without too much abnormality and this had always been most difficult. He visited his girl in Grand Rapids and talked fluently with her parents. About this time, however, he became anxious about financing his education in the fall. Working only four hours a day was not giving him enough money to make it through two semesters. He asked me what to do, and I told him he should decide. After several days of ambivalence which was reflected in his speech, he finally began to work in the factory from three to midnight. Often with overtime he would come to our conferences groggily, and he was unable to work as hard on his speech as he had before. Nevertheless, he adapted to the new schedule and held most of his gains. I suggested that he work on his speech and have a conference with me every other day so that he could sleep longer, but he disagreed. He still had things to do, he said.

For the first two weeks in August, I left the farm to give some lectures on the West Coast and to catch a fish in Alaska. When I returned, Don presented me with a set of daily reports for that period. He had continued to work but had not made any further progress. He had had a couple of rather poor days just before I came home. He was glad to see me. His speech was fast and cluttered at times but overall it was still pretty good except for the presence of miniature tremors and jaw jerks. "I'd like to ask a favor," he said in our first conference. "I've only got two more weeks before I leave the farm and go back to school. I'm doing all right, but there's still too much junk in my speech, and I don't know how to get rid of it. It's like the crud in the bottom of a jug. How do you get it out? Give me a suggestion, won't you?" I looked him over pretty closely and decided the plea was not for dependency but for professional advice. So I acceded.

I suggested that he schedule different periods of silence as a penalty contingent upon the type of residual stuttering behavior. Tremors with eye closings and jaw jerks were to be followed by a thirty second silence; tremors with jaw jerks alone, 20 seconds; tremors with smooth releases, 5 seconds of contingent silence. I gave him a card on which to type this sentence to show to any listener who became impatient: "I'm trying to overcome my stuttering and must be silent for a few seconds. Hope you don't mind." I also asked him to get a Polaroid snapshot made of his face in a very severe faked block of the old variety and to hold it in his hand and look at it during the silent penalty.

Don was appalled at the prospect. "That's crazy and unreasonable," he protested. I told him he didn't have to do it, but he had asked for a suggestion, and I had given him one. At our next conference he reported he had followed the schedule only a few times and suspected his moments of silence were not long enough even then and that he could not bear to look at the photo. I reflected his feelings and made no attempt to convince him to give it a real trial. He watched me very closely, then said, "You're an old devil!"

The next day he was jubilant. He had used the program during the whole day and his speech was wonderful. "It's clean," he said. He was speaking carefully but easily, and I heard or saw no sign of any stuttering whatsoever. He also had gone without lunch and had rewarded himself for every five sentences of good speech with a piece of chocolate until he was through work at midnight. He applied the reinforcement schedules rigorously for the rest of that week and here are some excerpts from his reports:

Speech-wise I had a very good day. It was very controlled and voluntary speech, and it was this way in most situations.
I was able to apply the reinforcement schedule quite effectively. The Hersheyettes are a very good token reinforcement, especially if I am quite hungry. At work I tried transfering a penny whenever I did a good job. Unfortunately, I didn't find this method as rewarding as the candy, even though I was able to buy an extra roll with it. Chances are one of the reasons the pennies didn't have as much reinforcement value was I would probably have eaten that extra roll anyway, since I worked quite late. The most satisfying thing about the transfering of pennies was the satisfaction I gained at the moment from being able to transfer a penny. Maybe

the physical act of transfering a penny helped to strengthen this satisfaction, but still the basic reinforcement was the knowledge that I did a good job.

I made calls to a couple of departments over at school as well as several other calls. I went to Sears where I had a couple of conversations with people there. I found out that most of the complaints that people had written the BROWN AND GOLD about were already solved, and I went down on the Mall and into Gilmores. My speech during these situations was quite good. At work I had two situations in talking to my bosses where I did not put in enough negative reinforcement, but otherwise I was quite pleased with how things went.

In all of the situations I am finding that both the demand to control myself and the realization that I am making real progress are both growing. There were a couple of times at work where after a situation I could not have handled too well a week ago and hardly at all three months ago, I felt like shouting, "Hey, listen to me! Aren't I doing a good job?" A very satisfying feeling.

Today I still had a lot of fear and anxiety about listener reaction if I would bring my card out. All morning long I dreaded pulling that card out. In fact, I dreaded it so much that my speech was so good that I didn't have to. I had a real good day as far as my speech was concerned.

I changed the program around some in order to make it easier to work with. Upon review I still find that it isn't what it should be. I have set too high penalties for my uncontrolled tremors with quick releases. Because the penalties are so severe, I refuse to subject myself to them. My program is attached.

My main speaking times during the morning were at the library, down at the Art Center, and a long conversation with the secretary of the First Congregational Church. During all of these conversations my speech was quite good with only a very few of the mild uncontrolled tremors. At work I had a number of the moderate uncontrolled releases as well as a lot of feared words that had a wobbly beginning.

After work I went to that company meeting where after seeing the slides, I had a good chance to talk during the refreshment period that followed. The conversation I enjoyed the most was when I was talking to the Detroit area salesman. I had a number of small blocks but I was able to apply the proper reinforcement schedule. There was one time when I should have probably brought the card out but I didn't. This was with a "bad" uncontrolled release.

I also had a conversation with a man down at Bronson Park, and one with a man down on the Mall. Both of these went really well.

At work I have begun to tell the guys what I am doing. I think this will help to structure the situation so that I will be able to better apply myself.

I allowed myself candy only after an entire conversation yesterday morning. This was because the situations that I was in made it impossible to eat in front of the person. I did have coffee with the church secretary, so that helped. If I had been thinking I could have used the refreshment period at work to my advantage.

All in all, quite a good day.

I had expected that some regression might occur during the last week before Don moved back to town, but this did not occur. He spoke very well in all situations, and there was none of the little repetitions or miniature blockings that had characterized his previous periods of better fluency. He was speaking easily but some evidence of proprioceptive monitoring was present. Don confessed he hated to leave but felt quite ready to do so, even eager to get back to college. "I feel about five inches taller when I go through a doorway," he said. "I'm not as scared as I thought I'd be at this point. Guess it's because I've really been on my own for two months and know what to do. I'll have some trouble probably, but I just can't conceive ever going back to the old stuff."

We saw him twice during the month that followed his departure. He is living with three other fellows in an old house and having fun. "I've almost forgotten what it means to be a stutterer. It's easy to talk now. Sometimes I talk too fast, but I know it and then speak more consciously." He enrolled in a discussion class in the speech department and participated with eagerness and complete fluency, his instructor reported. He made a speech before a seminar in speech pathology for an hour without any signs of stuttering. His girl says he is cured.

We shall see.

transcript from tape prepared by Don for the period
August 30—November 15

The Sunday before school began, I moved out of the apartment at Dr. Van's farm and moved into a house with three other guys. I was rather apprehensive about this move and about starting back to school because of all the new pressures as well as all the old pressures which would be there. I think it was the old pressures that I was especially worried about. I guess I didn't think I might be able to hold up and maintain the new type of speaking once I got back into the swing of things and started the old grind.

However, the first week was very rewarding. It was probably the most enjoyable week I've ever had in my life, especially in school. I was almost intoxicated with my speech, and the feeling of being able to ask questions easily in class, to give my name, talk to friends, do things like that. I spoke like that for over three weeks, and I guess I got a little speech-drunk. I talked all the time. And then I started to let the little blocks, the little tremors, the little avoidances get by. But for that month I was able to maintain a very good level of fluency. I did notice that my speech was beginning to get faster, and I believe I started to lose my proprioceptive monitoring and my voluntary speech.

I had found my classwork full of speaking situations. Both Dr. Van and I had felt that it would be very worthwhile for me to take a speech course, so I signed up for a four hour discussion course. Also, I had a course in Management Problems, which is basically a discussion course, and other courses like Auditing and Business Law and Economics. All these except for the law and business course were relatively small, so there was chance to talk a lot. I did.

About the fourth week, however, I hit a bad point. For about a week I went downhill very rapidly. I felt the relapse beginning with little sticky blocks like bbb-brown and Ddd-avid. I'd had some bouncy ones that first month and these weren't long ones, but they felt longer. Compared to what I had last spring they were relatively little ones. Not bad, really, but they began to bother me. Then I started avoiding some words and then some more and getting more apprehensive about it. These little surprising blocks came before the apprehension, but I could feel the fear begin to zoom. I tried to dodge them to protect my fine fluency or to ignore them. I knew I was getting worse.

And then I remember that the first panel I was on in Discussion Class came up on a Thursday, and the setback had started the previous weekend. The stuttering had kept getting worse, and the fear, until the night before the discussion, when I was really scared about it. Up to that point I had been eagerly looking forward to giving it because I felt I could do a good job, but that night before I was really scared. But the next day I gave it at 3:00 in the afternoon, and speechwise it went quite well. I was number seven on an eight man panel, so you can imagine the communicative stress that was building up, the anxiety and the fear. I felt like my stomach was going to fall apart on me because of the butterflies down there. But I gave it all I had, and fortunately I had a real strong beginning. I was able to maintain my composure and my voluntary speech. I guess I spoke much too fast, however; but as the blocks went, there weren't any that I noticed. Felt good. I was on top of it. Since then my speech has got much better and my fears have gone down. I'm talking pretty good for some time now, but I'm working on it again.

I think the things I'm learning now are: I must keep on top of those little blocks and avoidances and recognize them honestly. I must make some effort each day to analyze how well I've been doing and to make little assignments to take care of what is wrong. I must keep my speech as voluntary as possible. I think probably the most important thing was the first point of not letting anything get by, if at all possible. After a little block, I wait five or ten seconds, rehearse it so I know what I did, then say it right. I think at this point this cancellation is more important than it ever has been. It kind of puts a proper model right back in my memory core instead of leaving a bad stuttering model in there; it erases it. Also, one thing we found this summer that is still useful is warm-up speech. I'm not doing this every day, but I try to do it at least a couple of times each week or more. I read to myself, feeling my good movements, and aloud and strong. I find this good to do early in the morning because I'm usually the only one up, and I study this way. Also, something else I think is very important is to scan situations ahead and analyze what pressures there are going to be and to figure out how to resist them.

I am still avoiding occasionally, really rather rarely, and I am still having some mild blocks, and once in awhile a big hard one when I'm off guard. In fact, just this Monday night I got stuck in a hard block. I followed my roommate over to campus. He has to park his car off campus, so I was going to give him a ride up to class. But I hadn't told him this. As his car pulled up alongside mine, I opened the door, and of course he was on the other side of his car and because of the hurry or something, that block happened. I hadn't expected it at all, but I jerked it out and think I made a face. Things like this are happening once in a while when I'm caught by surprise. Also I have trouble on my name and things like that. But they don't petrify me now. I guess I would prefer having these right now, little and big, than being completely fluent and then having them hit me in say, six months or a year from now. They're good reminders that I have some way to go before becoming a good speaker, but I think I'm well on my way.

I might say that all in all I feel good. I got through that little relapse without help and all by myself. My speech is pretty good; not as good as I want it to be or as it will be someday, but it's like a miracle compared with how it was. I have to talk in my job as editor of the BROWN AND

GOLD. The phone's always ringing; one problem after another. I have to talk continuously, and a lot of speaking is in situations where I had a terrible time last year. Now it's easy. I almost forget how it was. I'm doing O. K., Doc. Van.

November 15—December 18

During this period, Don made marked progress. He made excellent grades including an A in his Discussion course. His instructor called me to tell me how well he had done, that he had made better contributions and was more poised and fluent than most of the others, that his final oral presentation, a solo effort, was masterful.

Don has evidently felt no need to see me. He had planned to have dinner with us this last week but phoned to say that he had an invitation to go to his girl's house then and would it be all right with us if he took a snowcheck. I took the opportunity to talk to him at some length and to review his last month. He had promised to make another taped report but said he was just too busy. He said his speech was very, very good though he still had an occasional short block (which he cancelled) when caught off guard or surprised. I noticed no sign of stuttering though he spoke with a bit more strength than before, and slower. He said he did not avoid at all but had a few weak fears at times. He says he's O.K. now.

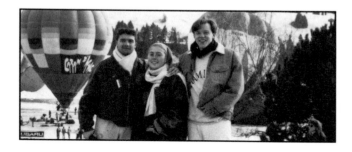

A CLINICAL FAILURE: MELINDA
CLINICIAN: C. VAN RIPER

I have had a number of stutterers with whom I have consistently failed despite strenuous efforts to help them. They seem to me to have some characteristics in common, and the person I have called Melinda is quite representative of this group. At the termination of therapy, they were stuttering as frequently and severely as they were at its beginning. Follow-ups were difficult to achieve, but in those I was able to contact several years later, the disorder showed no change. Repeatedly I have reviewed their case folders and my clinical notes to try to comprehend the reasons for their intransigence or my ineptitude. Perhaps this analysis will be more successful than those which preceded it. Anyway:

Melinda, when she first enrolled in our program of intensive therapy, was a very attractive girl, one of the most beautiful girls I have known. She also stuttered more consistently and with greater frequency than almost any stutterer I have met. On the average about 90% of her words showed abnormality and this frequency rate did not vary much from situation to situation. Though occasionally she might say a phrase or short sentence without repetitions, only once did I hear her be completely fluent for several minutes. Melinda was making a phone call and did not know anyone was near, and she was giving some girl friend billy blue hell. For almost five minutes she talked freely and with much profanity and vulgarity. When I walked in, her voice and speech changed, and the stuttering reappeared.

Melinda's stuttering was monosymptomatic, consisting of rapid syllabic repetitions using the schwa vowel. I once counted 28 on a single word with an inspiration taken partway through the sequence, but the number of repetitions closely averaged about seven or eight. Very few were less than three. She was the only stutterer I have ever heard to compulsively repeat the final unaccented syllable of a polysyllabic word. Often if by chance she would happen to say several words in a row without stuttering, I would hear her return to the phrase or last word thereof and repeat its first or accented syllable. She cancelled her fluent words by stuttering.

Another characteristic of the repetitions was the lack of accompanying tremors or fixations. They were not very regular in their tempo. They started slowly then became faster. Once started, they ran on, uninterrupted until the word was uttered. No rise in pitch accompanied the accelerating repetitions nor was there any tension or struggle. She just buh-buh-buh-buh-buh-bounced and bounced interminably. Interestingly enough, though she reported situation fears, she had few phonemic or word fears. Melinda could not remember the sounds of words on which she had stuttered even though I requested an accounting immediately after the conclusion of an utterance. A seeming detachment (or a real one) existed which apparently insulated her from the confrontation of her abnormal speech behavior. She could not sense it, remember it or stop it. When I placed a mirror before her, she shut her eyes or they became glazed. When I played back a recording, she would just laugh. "That sure sounds silly, doesn't it?" she said but without affect. I never could get Melinda to accept her stuttering objectively. She gaily and easily admitted that she was a stutterer, in fact "a stuttering mess" but the comment always seemed perfunctory.

Melinda showed very few avoidances. She entered all ordinary speaking situations, telephoned, interrupted, argued. She enrolled in several classes in public speaking much to the distress of her instructors. One of them told my "My god, keep those stutterers out of my hair. That Melinda girl tortures all of us. She takes up more class time than any three other students combined. If she weren't as sweet and beautiful and courageous, I'd kick her out."

Melinda showed few postponement tricks antecedent to her repetitions, no "ah's" or "uhms" as starters, no circumlocution or substitutions. She plunged directly into her repetitive utterance without any sign of faltering. Another characteristic, perhaps significant, was that she showed no reaction immediately after her moments of stuttering, no pauses, no flushing, nothing. The basic prosody was unaffected except for reduced inflection. She spoke a stuttering language.

Melinda always maintained excellent eye contact. She had beautiful jet black eyes, and she kept them upon you constantly, almost hypnotically. She seemed always to be scanning you—testing, testing, testing. The intensity of her gaze increased at the moments of stuttering. At the same time, however, she smiled, a bittersweet smile. Not much humor it it—just a beautiful, brave little girl smiling away the monsters and ghosts. Most people did not see her testing eyes—only her smile—and Melinda had, in fact, received very few consistent penalties for her stuttering. She always seemed to have girl friends and acquaintances in quantity though the relationships seemed unstable. Melinda's brave little smile reduced others into wanting to mother or take care of her. "She seems so brave and sweet" one of her housemothers said. I found Melinda as tough as Naugahyde and hard as corundum.

She was not helpless at all. She was one of the most controlling females I have ever met—and that constitutes more than a covey. Even her whims were iron.

In the course of my career I have come to expect resistance from my clients as part of the therapy process—indeed as a very essential part. Too much compliance always worries me. Anyone who has stuttered for years has incorporated the disorder into the very bones of his personality. There is rendering of soul flesh when one begins to remove it. We protect and seek to maintain all equilibria even those uncomfortable ones which distress us. But Melinda fought me to the ground whenever I sought to get her to modify her stuttering. Very intelligent, she constantly outwitted me. To cite but one example, once I had contrived to get her to promise to appear before a group of speech therapists at a professional meeting and to describe and comment upon each moment of stuttering she experienced. She was committed. I had blocked—so I thought—every other exit. I took her to the meeting in my car. Five minutes before the meeting after going to the ladies' room she told me she could not go through with it. Her face was covered with a reddist purple rash; her eyes were almost swollen shut. Even her arms and hands were puffed and discolored. All that had happened in five minutes. I surrendered then as I often had before and kicked myself for my stupidity in hoping that finally she had been brought to the point of accepting her stuttering as a problem.

As I look back on all those daily sessions (and I worked with her daily for a year) I wonder why I persisted. It was probably professional vanity. I had come to have the illusion that I was a pretty good therapist with stutterers. Melinda and her ilk have taught me professional humility. I now think she enjoyed the whole business. She played the game skillfully, always giving me enough intermittent hope to allow the game to continue. I believe she knew she would win. She played games with me. Were they sexual games? If so, she covered the dynamics skillfully. Certainly there was no sign of flirtation in her behavior. Could it have been a latent homosexuality, using the therapy room as the battlefield against a male therapist? Melinda dated several boys regularly and evidently enjoyed them, and they her. I interviewed one of the boys who had taken her out repeatedly, and he said she was fun but not very hot. "I always have the feeling she's watching herself and me. She's not there." For two months I administered therapy through an attractive woman therapist. No difference.

In my review of her file, I find that my clinical notes on our therapy sessions are sketchy, much more so than those of the other stutterers I have served. In part this was due to the fact that Melinda revealed very little about herself despite my probings. She was an incredibly expert conversational fencer. Her lie score on the MMPI was high, and I never really trusted any information she offered. I know that she often did not tell the truth about her self therapy assignments. In our sessions together, however, she was usually quite cooperative in a token way, always doing a little but never enough. At times she would report a glorious triumph in a situation which I could never check upon. A few "facts" may be given here. Melinda was an only child of wealthy parents. Very precocious physical and social development. Began to stutter suddenly on school entrance into kindergarten at five years. Stuttering was severe and frequent from the first. "My parents tell me it's the same now as it was then." No stuttering in the family. A pleasant home. The usual summer camps and travels. Excellent education achievement. Accepted socially despite her stuttering. Parents had sought all sorts of professional help and "finally, they just gave up on me" she reported. Melinda had her own car at college, plenty of money and dressed attractively.

The reader of this little piece will of course be wondering why I accepted such a case for speech therapy or continued to work with her for two years. I do not think it was just because she was beautiful but rather because that her stuttering was so consistent and frequent. No one should have to go through life talking like that. All the patterning of behaviors indicated neurosis and I recognized this very soon, but I have always considered the particular kind of speech therapy I practice to be essentially a psychotherapy, too. Most severe stutterers show signs of neurosis, though, it is usually an expectancy neurosis. Melinda could not be described as phobic in any stretch of the word. She had very little expectancy. I could find no evidence of profit from her symptoms though possibly they might serve as a defense against a latent homosexuality. To check this, I referred Melinda to a psychiatrist colleague for whom I have the profoundest respect. After a series of interviews, he assured me that no primary neurosis existed. Also Melinda told me that a famous psychoanalyst in Boston had explored the matter for several months and had refused to accept her for deep analysis saying that she did not need it. It is my feeling now that Melinda fooled them, too. Perhaps I am merely trying to salvage my own professional self respect, but I'm pretty well convinced that her stuttering was symptomatic of a deep primary neurosis. When finally I confessed my inability to continue therapy for another single session and confronted her with this diagnosis, Melinda said with that same brave, sweet smile, "Oh, I'm sorry too, Dr. Van. I had such hopes in you. But please, Dr. Van, you must not let this experience make you feel incompetent or discouraged." Damn her hide!

A CLINICAL SUCCESS: JOHN
CLINICIAN: DEAN E. WILLIAMS

introduction

In order to select a client with whom I believe I succeeded, it was necessary to establish certain criteria as to what one means by success. A case was selected for whom there was a complete typed transcript of the therapy sessions, and upon review of these transcripts, I believe I maintained (1) consistency of overall philosophy, (2) consistency of purpose, (3) sensitivity to what the client was attempting to communicate to me, and (4) logicalness of the principles and procedures emphasized. At the termination of therapy, the client was speaking essentially normally in all speaking situations (one syllable repetitions occurred infrequently). Furthermore, he maintained or improved his speech behavior with the passage of time.

the case of John

John was a 24-year-old college graduate who had been working for his father since he graduated from college at the age of 21. He was single. He was a severe stutterer—he received a severity rating of six on a seven-point scale. He used a good many starters such as "I mean," "let's see," or "you see." His stuttering behavior consisted of very rapid, tense jaw movement with protrusion of tongue, head jerking, eye closure and excessive saliva forming around his mouth. At times it trickled down his chin. The tensing behavior extended throughout the body with particular tensing and movement of the hands and arms during any stuttering behavior.

He had received a year and a half of therapy at the speech and hearing clinic while he was attending college. This therapy consisted primarily of "working on an objective attitude, studying and controlling his blocks, etc." He reported that he felt the therapy helped him feel better about himself but that he had had little success in improving the ways he talked.

He reported that he began to stutter when he was three or four years old. He was an only child. From his report (and subsequently confirmed by meeting his parents), his mother was an extremely kind, over-protective mother who "felt" her child had a terrible handicap and she had to "run interference for him" during the time he was growing up. His father, on the other hand, was an extremely successful man both politically and in business. He was an out-going, socially acceptable aggressive individual who was very proud of his ability to meet people and to speak well. He was extremely concerned about the kind of future John would have in business when he had such difficulty in speaking.

John was seen for a total of 37 one-hour sessions. This was distributed over an eight-week period. In addition, he attended a group meeting for two one-hour sessions per week.

The therapy program began with the clinician inquiring about the kinds of problems John felt he had in getting along with other people and the nature of his attitudes and feeings that he believed created problems for himself. John began talking about his inability to solve problems in his daily living. He was concerned that he often felt he did not know the "right" things to do. He would vacillate between several alternative solutions toward most problems that arose. It took him considerable time to try to arrive at a "right" answer and by this time often he would decide there was little need to do anything about it. As a result, he felt guilty about his tendency to procrastinate on decisions and in meeting problems which tended to arise. He demonstrated the same kinds of indecision in trying to select a vocation. He was unhappy working for his father and yet he could not decide what else he wanted to do. As a result, he went unhappily to work each morning and returned each evening vowing he was going to have to decide soon on a vocation. He discussed problems he had with his money, with his automobile, etc. He resented the speed with which most boys his age, and especially his father, could arrive at a reasonable solution to their own problems—and to his problems when he explained them.

The clinical program began from this background. I adopted the role of a person who would attempt to help him become the kind of person who could solve his own problems. We began by taking some of his problems other than speech and began to discuss how one begins to employ a problem-solving approach. This included such things as (1) the difference between describing and evaluating, (2) trying to find the "right" solutions to problems versus attempting to first clearly define the questions, (3) thinking of all the different alternatives one has, (4) thinking of the consequences of each, and then (5) arriving at the most reasonable and practiced solution— with a willingness to pay the consequences for that decision. This involved a discussion of what is meant by a question. That is, the kinds of questions which could never be answered versus the kinds of questions which could be answered by discussion, reading, and experimentation. Finally, we discussed within the problem-solving attitude the necessity of "getting involved," of *acting upon* obtained information as opposed to an intellectual "game playing" with the information obtained.

The clinician adopted a role of helping him define the questions, of helping him learn the difference between a meaningful question and a "nonsense" question, of helping him define the different alternatives and then discussing with him the possible consequences. This was followed by adopting a role of providing emotional support for him as he cautiously adopted one course of action in relation to a problem and fearfully proceeded on it. The expression of feelings was encouraged as this decision-making procedure took place. Following this, the clinician asked the client questions, the most important of which was, how can you find out? Does one need to read and obtain information, does one need to discuss the problems with someone or can one go out and experiment by behaving in different ways and observing the consequences?

He brought up many topics for discussion with a request for help in learning methods for solving them. These included such items as dating, budgeting money, etc.

From the philosophy described above, it was easy to lead him into a discussion of the problems he encountered while talking, the ways he felt about them—and procedures for solving them. The ground work was laid that permitted him *to begin to see* that his job was to *change* his talking behavior and not one of "to stop stuttering."

It is not the purpose of this paper to discuss the therapy program emphasized in detail. The concepts discussed in therapy will be presented here only to the extent to which they illustrate the role which the clinicial played—and how the client responded.

John was able to observe his talking in a mirror and listen to it on a tape recording in order to begin to ask questions about what he could do about it. He observed in detail the process of normal speaking. We sat and read together so that he could observe the feeling and movement involved in talking. He then tried to duplicate the behavior involved in his stuttering behavior and to describe the difference between it and normal talking. I began to make assignments for him. These assignments were undertaken not to learn any "skill" but rather to make observations of his behavior—to learn from his own behavior. Basic to all of this was the question of how one can change these ways of acting.

He soon began to make his own assignments. What is more important, he set no specific number of assignments to do on any one day. Instead, he did the number of assignments which he had to do in order to learn what he was tying to learn. With this kind of approach to the clinical situation, he came to think of himself as an experimenter. It then became quite easy for him to change his ways of thinking from "what is my stuttering," to "what am I doing to interfere with talking," to "what do other people do when they talk?" He began to smooth out his talking process, to move forward in the talking process, to increase spontaneity, to tolerate feelings of fear and to recognize them as such while he went ahead and did things to talk.

The point I am trying to make is, with the relationship we had established, with the problem-solving attitude which John developed, I am not sure of the part I played after he began changing his talking behavior. He was excited by every change he made—because he was the one who was doing it. He came less to rely on me and more and more to rely on his own imagination and ingenuity in dreaming up kinds of situations where he could learn something about the ways he felt and the ways his feelings would change as he talked to people. He became extremely intrigued with the feelings that he called "anticipation." He became very confident in his ability to change his speaking behavior when he found that his "feelings of anticipation" would change as he changed the ways he was talking.

During this process, we discussed many items such as his relationship with his father, with his mother, the kind of business activities that he wished to engage in. He approached these in a problem-solving way.

At the termination of therapy he was very confident that he could apply these same principles when he got back home. He was certain that he could continue with his new found ways of talking, of interacting with people, and of solving his problems.

I followed John for three years. During this time his speech continued to improve. Recently, he wrote that at this time he considers himself for all practical purposes to be a normal speaker. He is involved in several business activities, is highly successful in these activities, is now married and has one child.

It is important to report that at the termination of therapy I asked him to think about and to discuss with me those aspects of therapy that he felt were the most important to him. He reported with no hesitation that the turning point in therapy came the day he found he could change the way he *felt* by the way he *behaved*. As he said, "I found out that I didn't just have to stand and do what I felt I had to do—I guess that's when I first really believed that I didn't have to talk the way I talked." He continued to elaborate, but it is important I think that essentially *he attributed* his improvement to one crucial experience—or observation.

concluding comments

The task of evaluating factors which may have contributed to success with John is not easy. The points which one considers important to the interaction are, of necessity, dependent upon ones own evaluations of what *he* considers "after the act" to have been related. However, it is my impression that several factors in relation to my role as a clinician are worthy of mention. First, we began with *his* definition of his problems, those things that were bothering him in getting along with other people and with himself. He learned how to solve these problems in ways other than on an emotional—

or an "I feel like it" level. He then was able to apply these same principles to his talking behavior so that the therapy procedures "made sense" to him.

It should be pointed out, however, that the above analysis was made after a careful review of typed transcripts of all therapy sessions. I must admit that at the time he terminated therapy I attributed much of the success to the "effectiveness" of the therapy techniques and to the ways assignments were made. This is important to mention because it was with this belief that I began to work with my next client named Susan. The therapy program with Susan is described elsewhere in this book as "a clinical failure."

A CLINICAL FAILURE: SUSAN
CLINICIAN: DEAN E. WILLIAMS

introduction

The selection of a client with whom I "failed" required certain decisions. I was tempted to select one whom I felt did not improve his speaking behavior to any great extent, but one for whom I felt I did everything possible. It has become obvious to me that by the time a person gets to be an adult there are some who do not appear to be "helpable." They do not benefit much from therapy. They appear to work to a fair degree on their speech, but they do not learn much—they just go through the motions of becoming involved in the therapy process with little change in their behavior. This occurs even though I feel I have done a satisfactory job as a clinician. There are other clients who fail for whom I feel I know where I "goofed." These are difficult to talk about because, as one unravels the story, certain "goofs" become very obvious and it appears they could have been avoided easily. This is particularly true if one has a typed transcript of all therapy sessions to review as I did.

I have selected the case of Susan. She represents a client who was "helpable." To me, she represents a failure because of my own errors in clinical judgment. It is a lesson I have never forgotten. It is presented with the hope it may help others.

the case of Susan

Susan came to the clinic accompanied by her husband. Her husband explained that the evening before they came to the clinic Susan began to cry and told him how much her speech bothered her. He stated they had been married for a year and a half and during that time she had never mentioned her speech. He stated that he was aware she stuttered slightly at times, but that she appeared so calm about it he never thought it bothered her. As a result, it had never been discussed during the year and a half of marriage or during the time they went together prior to marriage.

Susan was an attractive, quiet, dependent young lady. She was 22 years old. She reported she was happy that she was married and considered herself very lucky to have such a kind and considerate husband. She had had no previous therapy. She was seen for a total of 64 one-hour sessions spread over a nine-month period.

I began to work with Susan immediately after the extremely successful experience with John (reported earlier in this book). Unfortunately, I began therapy with the preconceived idea of what it was *I* wanted her to accomplish. There was no attempt to first find out what she considered to be her problems and then to begin at this point. In other words, I did not bother to *listen* to what she was trying to tell me. I was too busy explaining the "stuttering problem" and the therapy procedures she was to follow. (These therapy procedures were those employed with John, described elsewhere.) In spite of lecturing to students many times about the fallacy of treating all clients alike, I fell into the same trap. Early in therapy she made many attempts to tell me what the problems consisted of, but I did not listen. Susan stated that she began to stutter so far as she could remember before she began school. She was sure no one in her family could tell me any more about it because not too many knew she had a problem. She covered up by not talking very much. If she doubted her ability to say a word she either substituted or did not say anything. When she was asked to read in class she mumbled and for the most part "got by." Throughout high school she reported most generally she was able "to hide it," so people could not see it —but that "she felt it!"

She had two brothers and one sister. She wrote and told her sister that she was coming for therapy. She showed me the letter her sister wrote to her in response. Her sister was surprised she was receiving therapy because even though she had noticed that Susan stuttered, she did not think it bothered Susan much.

Early in therapy she attempted on many occasions "to tell me" that she was concerned and worried about her self-worth. Following are some examples from the transcript.

While obtaining a case history the following conversation took place: Clinician: "Do either of your brothers or your sister have a speech problem?" Susan: "No, they're all very sharp. I'm the failure of the family." Clinician: "Do you feel that way because of your speech?" Susan: "Not entirely."

I never pursued the point. I went on to inquire about when people first noticed that she had a problem and what anyone had ever said about it. In later therapy sessions while discussing her stuttering problem she said, "It's mental, I know it, I know it!" Instead of perceiving that she was reflecting a feeling—a fear, I began to discuss with her the vagueness and meaninglessness of thinking of stuttering as being "mental." Later on she mentioned on several occasions, "I am an odd case," or "I'm an odd ball, huh?"

On one other occasion I asked her to read for me aloud. She stated, "I might—in fact I know—I will be able to read perfectly, but I'm not perfect, far from it!" It can be observed that she started out talking about speech and ended up talking about herself. Again, I failed to perceive the point she was communicating. I went ahead by stating that no one is perfect—and no one can talk perfectly, and then proceeded to another point.

On another occasion the following conversation took place:

Clinician: "How has your speech been?"

Susan: "About the same."

Clinician: "How are you feeling about it?"

Susan: "I'm resigned to it."

Clinician: "Can you say anything more about that?"

Susan: "I'm not as nervous about it, but I hate (long pause) it just as much."

Here I left the point and went on to a discussion of how her speech was at the office (she was a secretary).

At another time in therapy the following conversation took place:

Susan: "The other day you mentioned that you were going to have me look in a mirror when I talk. I haven't done it yet."

Clinician: "We're going to do that one of these days."

Susan: "It must be a horrible sight. I don't want to do it. I don't like to look at myself in the mirror even when I don't stutter."

Again, I went on to something else.

The excerpts presented above are sufficient to illustrate the point I am trying to make. To review the transcripts was a demoralizing experience for me. Unfortunately, I did not review them until the termination of therapy. We were slow in getting the therapy sessions typed. By the time they were typed we were on some other point in therapy and, as such things go, "I never got around to it."

In studying the transcripts, it was noted that most of the comments mentioned above were made during approximately the first three months of therapy. From approximately the fourth month of therapy on to the end, at any time I began to inquire about or to discuss the ways she felt about herself, she would lead me off in a different direction. Unfortunately, on every occasion I went along with her. This also was the approximate time in therapy when she began to make "progress" on her speech. She became increasingly active in working on her speech, in discussing attitudes about *stuttering*, and in talking about her interactions with other people (related to *stuttering*). It appeared as if she decided to go along with me on speech and attitudes about speech because it enabled her to avoid discussing things which were relatively more painful. Also, I imagine that as I directed the therapy sessions, she became more and more resigned to "the procedure one follows in working on stuttering." She became quite cooperative—and even determined. She began to carry out all of her assignments. She began to test her attitudes and feelings about *stuttering*. She began to discuss her speech with other people. And, she showed steady improvements in fluency. She became interested in reading about the problem of stuttering. She became familiar with some of the writings of various people in the profession. One point which came out was the discussion of heredity in relation to the cause of stuttering. She confessed one day that she was scared to have any children because she was afraid they may stutter. By providing information and through discussions she came to see this fear as being unrealistic.

She reached a point where she was talking very well in all situations. In fact, it was nearing the time when her husband was going to leave school and move to another town and she was very happy about the wohle thing. She was most appreciative of the "tremendous help" that she received from me.

A month after she left the clinic I received a letter from her that her "speech had utterly and completely collapsed." She reported that she was much worse than she had been for years. She reported that she was horrified by it and could not bear to go out of the house to meet anybody because of the terrible impression it would leave on the friends of her husband. He was beginning a new job and she was afraid that she would hold him back. She requested an appointment to see me. She drove 280 miles to have a conference. Prior to this conference I studied the clinical transcripts for hours. Much of what is reported to you became dreadfully obvious. When she appeared for her conference we talked over the problems that we had not discussed previously. She disintegrated into tears. She admitted that she viewed herself as a very inadequate person. She was fearful that she could never be a good wife and mother. She always had felt that whenever she stuttered it told people that she was a "very defective person." She went on to relate that by working to improve her speech she hoped she could get to a point where other people could not see how "inadequate" she was even though she still felt it inside. She agreed to seek help in the town in which she now lived. Fortunately, there was a clinician available in that area. I called the individual, sent excerpts from the transcript, and pointed out as best I could where I had "goofed" in therapy.

She began a therapy program in which she worked to face herself—to understand the problem in relation to her feelings about herself as a person. They evaluated her concept of herself and slowly she came to view herself in a much more healthy perspective. It is interesting to note that as this took place she picked up and began to implement direct speech changes which she had learned in therapy and soon reached the point where she terminated therapy on her own account. I since have heard from her on many occasions. She reports that she is talking fine, that she wants to have five children, and at this time has two. Her husband is getting along fine. She is active in community activities.

To date, it looks like a happy ending. It is obvious, however that the happy ending came about in spite of a serious clinical error made on my part.

PART II

Notes From The Conference Discussions

The descriptions of successes and failures reveal many things about our therapies for stutterers—and about ourselves as clinicians. Perhaps they reveal more than we wish you to see! Certainly the case studies could stand alone, but as we each read them, questions arose, fervent discussions ensued, and we felt we had many important insights about the fascinating and puzzling process called therapy.

But how do you report in a meaningful fashion a six-day flow of words from ten individuals experienced and interested in therapy with stutterers? There were the challenging and demanding questions—"Why did you do that?", "How did you know what to do and when to do it?" "What makes you think you had that influence on the stutterer—wasn't it something within the stutterer himself?"—and so on. At times we wanted to get up on a soapbox and expound a whole philosophy of living; at other times, we were amazingly patient listeners. Occasionally, penetrating and brilliant comments were made, accepted as such, and then lost in the welter of new ideas that branched off from them. Always, we eventually returned to the central core of questions and ideas around which the conference was organized—the relationship of the clinician to the therapeutic process.

The notes or generalizations which are presented below constitute a sampling of some of the ideas that emerged during the week of discussion. As such, they fall far short of expressing the dynamic character of the ideas or the exciting interaction among the participants. They only partially reflect the complex unity of the concepts. In spite of our difficulty in translating these insights into words, we hope they may prove stimulating.

varying criteria for success and failure

The conference first came to grips with its titled agenda. What did we mean by success and failure? Successes and failures are not to be viewed solely as terminal absolutes. They both occur in miniature in every session. They always occur. They may summate or cancel each other. Today's failure may encapsulate the seeds of tomorrow's success and the reverse of this proposition also is true. What is vitally important is that the clinician should be highly aware of any discrepancies between his own and the stutterer's definitions of success or failure since these probably affect the final outcome.

In general we would say that the criteria of success and failure will vary with each stuttering problem and perhaps with each therapist. Some of our claimed successes may continue to stutter to some degree; we are not so perfectionistic as to insist upon perfection. The question we asked ourselves was this: Did we truly help this stutterer to communicate much more effectively and to live with comparative ease in a verbal world?

the initial relationship between client and clinician

As the participants studied the case histories, it became apparent that many of the seeds of success—and of failure—were sown early in the therapy relationship. We tried to pinpoint some of the factors that occurred early in the therapeutic sessions and that seemed to be related to eventual success.

belief in eventual success.

Both the stutterer and the clinician must have a conviction that success is possible. Each may have his own sources for this faith. The stutterer may have faith in the basic competence of the clinician, even if it is simply an appreciation that what the therapist proposes to do in therapy makes sense. The clinician derives confidence from his basic understanding of people, his understanding of stuttering as a disorder, and from his experience with other stutterers. He recognizes that a primary problem is to find successive steps of the right size that will insure a progression to the desired goals. Furthermore, the faith of the stutterer and the clinician are interactive. It is important for the clinician to be viewed as someone who understands enough to help the stutterer to do what he thinks he cannot do. It is equally important for the stutterer to be viewed by the clinician as someone who has the ability to change his problem. The interaction of this faith is an apparent necessity for successful therapy.

the clinician as seen by the stutterer.

Initially, it seems important that the clinician be viewed as someone *unique*—as someone who is different from others the stutterer has known. As one participant, in analyzing his success with a child, stated, "He saw me as someone who was not going to manipulate him from the outside as others had." Perhaps the stutterer views the clinician at times as a "magic healer," as a person with special information, or simply as the first person who seemed to understand both him and his stuttering and is concerned and hopeful about his ability to solve the problem.

The wise clinician recognizes also that he is restricted to varying degrees in the roles he can present to the stutterer. Various factors such as his age, his position, his physical size and appearance, and his personality are relatively unchangeable and are a part of the total picture perceived by the client. For example, a clinician close to the generation of the stutterer can function in ways that are not available to the clinician who is noticeably older or younger than the stutterer. Awareness of such limitations may enable the therapist to use more effectively those roles which are available to him.

the stutterer as seen by the clinician.

In terms of the successes reported here, there seemed to be a relationship between success and the extent to which the clinician recognized some positive traits in the stutterer. We identified with the case or with his needs. Perhaps we were reacting to his potential for change. Certainly there appeared to be some kind of interaction at work that had a bearing on success.

"in the world and with it."

In describing Sherrie's father, Emerick artfully states that the father was "in the world but not of it." The reverse of this statement seemed to characterize the therapist's initial views of their success cases. Those who improved were aware of and still successfully involved in the world around them. This is not to say that the successful stutterers did not have problems, for many did. But, in general, the successful cases seemed to represent the "normalcy" end of the continuum despite their communication difficulties.

readiness to work.

A characteristic of most of the successful stutterers we studied was that they appeared to "go for yardage each time they got the ball." They exhibited a determination and even a certain amount of "recklessness" in the way they proceeded. They accepted the responsibility for doing something about their speech.

There were many examples of well-directed energy among those cases we considered successful. For example, Louise was the only member of her group who followed up on a suggested reading and appeared to benefit from it. Alex was described as one who challenged ideas and then was "reckless enough to take a chance and see what happened." Cora's therapist stated that she ". . . brought to therapy an analytic, rational attitude toward problems . . ."

Among the less successful, a few, such as Sherrie, appeared to desire to get involved but failed ever to do so. How much of this determination and energy is engendered by the clinician and how much is brought to therapy by the stutterer? Apparently, the clinician can encourage or even create this at times. Many of the participants felt that Don's dedicated application and willingness to do what was suggested was the direct result of the challenge set by his clinician. One suggestion for instilling a ready-to-work attitude among cases was to create some initial success of which the client is aware. For example, one participant reported that the quick modification of a particularly distressing secondary behavior apparently spurred one of his stutterers to engage energetically in other phases of therapy.

establishing a beneficial climate.

The importance of creating a relationship which allows the clinician to proceed with what he feels will result in success was brought out in several ways in the discussion of the cases. As the clinician and the stutterer increase their understanding of each other, the therapeutic process moves forward. In some instances, failure was apparently due to the absence of this type of understanding relationship.

One approach for improving the initial relationship between the stutterer and the clinician is for the latter to attempt to recognize the level of understanding and the value system of the stutterer. As clinicians we should not be content with providing help only for those whose personality and way of thinking match our own. Perhaps some of our failures would have been successes had we tried harder to understand the stutterers' belief system about his stuttering, about himself as he now is, and perhaps more importantly, about the kind of person he is striving to become.

Perhaps the most favorable therapeutic climate is created when the clinician perceives within the stutterer something of himself— a life, in part, that he has experienced. As the clinician finds ways to enlarge his own life experience, he undoubtedly becomes able to work successfully with more people who stutter.

the contract between stutterer and clinician.

One of the important features of success seems to be the existence and acceptance of what Meninger has termed "the contract." The clinician must first clarify what he will do and what he expects the stutterer to do. This clarification can take many forms and degrees of explicitness, but the basic element that should be made clear is that the clinician agrees to function in ways which he thinks will be helpful for the stutterer. With stutterers who have had no previous therapy, clarification may involve some explanation of the general process that is anticipated. With those who have had previous therapy, it may be important to explain differences in the approach to be employed. The stutterer somehow needs to recognize and demonstrate acceptance of his part of the contract. In some instances, particularly when the contract is made explicit, there may be a rapid and wholehearted acceptance of the contract on the part of the stutterer. At least, this seems to have been the pattern among most of our successful cases. Note, for example, the explicitness of the contract and the degree of acceptance indicated in the case study of Don.

But establishing the proper relationship or contract is frequently not an easy task. Many stutterers find it difficult to know how to function within the therapeutic relationship. Perhaps this is because their way of relating to others has been distorted by their speech problem. Sometimes the "rules" of the clinical relationship are so much more definite than in normal life. The clinician must understand these complexities and difficulties. To the stutterer, the therapy relationship is new, strange, and, perhaps, even threatening. It seems important that we, as clinicians, recognize this and structure therapy so that the client understands his responsibilities. It is equally important that we recognize the two-party nature of this contract and fulfill our part of the bargain.

setting the best course.

A frequently posed question during the meeting, and probably one which confronts all clinicians, went something like this: "Do you suppose I started off on the wrong track—did I emphasize the wrong aspect of therapy?" Certainly all clinicians are faced with choices about the direction for beginning therapy or the type of therapy to be initiated. Many cases have complex case histories. The problems they present are myriad. How can a clinician know whether to attack the "non-speech-related" aspects of the problem or to concentrate primarily upon the patient's stuttering. Susan's clinician felt that his major error was in not fitting therapy to certain primary needs. In the case of Louise and Alex, therapy moved well despite the fact that each of these people had many other problems which, during therapy, were not dealt with directly. How does the clinician know where to concentrate his efforts?

Several possible answers to this question were suggested. Some of the participants preferred a global approach, that is, a simultaneous attack on several problems. Others felt that the more basic problems should be cleared up before seeking to effect changes in speech behavior.

It seldom appears necessary to attend immediately to all of the stutterer's problems. It may be possible to rank these according to some criteria such as severity, obviousness, or importance, and to begin on the problem considered most critical. These may not necessarily coincide with what the patient thinks is most severe.

In some instances, particularly when the problems appear quite complex and other sources of help are not readily available, the therapist may limit therapy to the elements he feels most competent to handle. For example, he may decide to concentrate entirely upon changing the speech behavior. All the participants reported successes with such an approach, frequently with individuals who continued to give evidence of having other problems long after successful speech therapy. Also, instances were reported where there had been a significant reduction in non-speech related problems as a result of progress with speech.

Some participants reported using a speech-centered approach on a tentative basis to allow time for continued observation and judgment as to the necessity for therapy oriented toward the other problems. Certainly, many practical factors contribute to such therapy decisions. It seems important that we be conscious of any decision to approach or to avoid therapeutic challenges, that we recognize our reasons for this decision, and that we monitor the therapeutic process for any signs that a change in approach is needed.

"with the third ear."

We felt we would probably have had fewer questions about the necessity for attacking various problems had we followed Theodore Reik's advice and learned to "listen with the third ear" more often. A primary skill of the therapist should involve the ability to understanding what the stutterer is trying to communicate in all of his behaviors—both verbal and non-verbal. Many failures apparently arose from the clinician's lack of sensitivity to all of the common forms of communication. Perhaps we fail to allow the stutterer to present enough of his problem picture before beginning active therapy. Too often we ignore such communicators as the tone of his voice, the repetitiveness of topics, the intensity of expression, the postures and gestures, or the contradictory behaviors he exhibits. Through experience, we can learn the cues that signal a potential breakdown in the therapeutic relationship. For example, the stutterer starts to be late for appointments, he appears bored, he forgets or only partially does assignments after a history of having completed all of them, or we find ourselves doing all the talking. Some of the therapists at the conference suggested that our skill in reading this silent language could be increased by reviewing each therapy session soon after it occurs and asking ourselves questions about the nature of what the stutterer was actually trying to communicate. All of us do this to some degree, but too often it is left undone. A recent success may subtly lead the clinician to repeat the process with a subsequent individual even though it may be inappropriate. (For example, see the case studies of Susan and Alex.) The clinician's firm convictions—his system of beliefs about stuttering—may act as filters which limit or distort what he observes.

involvement of others in therapy.

In seeking to determine the basic course of therapy, a clinician is sometimes faced with the question of how much to involve other persons besides the stutterer in therapy. This question arises more frequently and seems to be more crucial when working with children. Perhaps it is well to say that, just as it is recognized that the stutterer is not the only member of the stuttering problem, the clinician should realize that he is not the only therapist. The younger the child, the more likely it is that the child's parents and teachers are significant parts of both the problem and the therapy. The successful clinician is he who learns to utilize each of the significant members of the problem to an optimum degree in correction of the problem. However, it is apparent that some parents have difficulty in accepting their responsibilities in this respect. At times, it may be necessary to create a subculture within the clinic in which the child's family is not included as a way of bringing about change. When the stutterer makes significant improvement without the family's help, their perception of the child and his problem is frequently altered, and they may become better able to cooperate effectively in therapy. Something like this appeared to occur in the case of Mark. After the clinician had initiated changes through application of a paternal role, the father changed his perception of his son and became able to establish a healthy relationship with him.

stutterer-clinician relationships during the course of therapy

All experienced clinicians recognize that there is much more to therapy than establishing initial rapport. Therapy is continual interaction. The therapist does not decide upon one role and then never change. The clinician's behavior is modified by what the stutterer does—how he reacts—etc. The therapist may need to be a stern taskmaster at one stage in therapy and a kind, understanding, tolerant friend at another. As the speech pathologists attending this conference examined their successes and failures, they came to realize that some of the problems encountered were difficulties in role adjustment during therapy.

One of the participants pointed out that the interpersonal interaction between clinician and stutterer during the course of therapy may vary along a continum ranging from a focus on the stutterer's affect (feelings, inspiration, support, etc.) to a focus on "things to do" (goals, assignments, etc.). More often than not, we find ourselves attempting to widen our perceptual lenses wide enough to focus on both feelings and activities.

problems in moving to a new relationship.

It is one thing to recognize that role changes are necessary and another to know when and how to make such changes. How can a clinician know, for example, when to shift from a focus on feelings to techniques of behavior modification? Many experienced clinicians include some exploratory testing in almost every session. For example, during the time the therapist is establishing a relationship that encourages the stutterer to express his feelings, he provides brief opportunities for the stutterer to test the attitudes in life situations. Depending on the client's reactions, the clinician may have the stutterer move ahead into a new stage or he may decide to back up and wait for awhile before changing the emphasis of therapy of the type of interaction already established.

the effects of the stutterer on the clinician.

Too frequently the clinical role is discussed only in terms of the clinician upon the stutterer. It seems reasonable, however, to recognize that some of the success of a clinician is, in part, a reflection of how the stutterer affects the clinician. One common element was apparent in most of the successes reported—the stutterer demonstrated in some way that he accepted the value system of the clinician, thus reinforcing the clinician's behavior in directions which proved to be salutory. Conversely, the failure did not seem to stimulate the therapist to beneficial responses. For example, some of us recognized that we have been made to feel fairly successful by the case's appeal to specific needs or weaknesses that we have. We all have gaps in our armour. Some of us seem to be peculiarly vulnerable to those who look on us as a possible Savior . . . or the oracle possessing all wisdom. Others fall victim to the stutterer who looks on us as a pleasant companion. We each have certain personal needs and weaknesses and so may allow a case's reaction to make us virtually impotent unless we are aware of these possibilities and guard against them.

limitations of a friendly relationship.

We generally accept the idea that success demands a very close relationship with stuttering cases. But as may be seen in Harry's case, too close a relationship, particularly when it is satisfying one of our personal needs, can prove detrimental to therapy. If we allow the therapy relationship to be dominated by friendliness, serious limitations in our effectiveness usually result. We may find we cannot motivate the stutterer to do what we think needs to be done. If the stutterer views therapy strictly as a friendly relationship, he may be reluctant to discuss feelings which he fears may threaten the friendship. None of this discussion should imply that the clinician should not be friendly with the stutterer, but our analysis of successes and failures indicated to us that when we allow a clinical relationship to satisfy our personal needs we tend to limit our ability to help the stutterer.

the problem of resistance in therapy

One of the topics of discussion that led to fervent interaction among the participants and to a good deal of honest soul searching concerned the apparent resistance of the stutterer. Whether an individual's failure to follow the therapist's lead in therapy is related to his own psychological needs or is a misperception on the part of the therapist is doubtlessly a moot question. The fact remains that, particularly among those whose therapy appears unsuccessful, the stutterer and his clinician did not appear to be on the same wavelength.

"Resistance" by the stutterer may take many forms, any one of which may be threatening to the clinician. The methods for dealing with resistance will need to vary with the basis for and the nature of the resistance. In general, it is well to respect resistance as evidence of some important need on the part of the stutterer. The stutterer may resist therapy simply because it demands work and change. His desire for homeostasis may be strong enough so that any change becomes threatening. He may be reacting to confused and inept approaches utilized by the therapist. And there are other reasons.

demands by the stutterer.

Some stutterers resist by demanding. Stutterers frequently make covert or overt demands upon the clinician. Some demands are a cry for help. Others are essentially infantile attempts to wrest control of the clinical process from the therapist—a way of manipulating or dominating him. These demands may be met or ignored, depending on which of these characteristics seem to be predominant in the judgment of the clinician. Conscious attention to their occurrence should aid us to become skilled in our clinical judgments.

Like many other problems, the dependency of the stutterer on the clinician is not to be regarded casually. We ought not to exploit our own needs by reinforcing dependency nor be unaware of the case's tendency to block therapeutic change by his unwillingness to accept personal responsibility. Temporary dependency is understandable and can be used constructively, but if such a relationship continues interminably, the potential of positive therapeutic change is greatly reduced.

reactions to little failures.

During the course of therapy, we all encounter times when stutterers fail in some assignment or sub-goal that has been planned. Just how we react to these small failures can be crucial in terms of the stutterer's eventual success or failure. Properly handled, failure can become a stimulant to increased growth and effort on the stutterer's part. Failure can sometimes be utilized to help a stutterer learn a better approach to problem-solving. On the other hand, an inappropriate reaction by the clinician can reinforce a sense of futility or an insufficient degree of effort by the stutterer.

expression of feelings by the therapist.

When a case displays resistance to therapy, we frequently must decide how and in what ways we should display or communicate our reactions. How can our own feelings be used to clarify the problem for the stutterer? Carl Rogers tells us he has found that a clinical relationship is not helped if the therapist tries to act loving when, at the moment, he feels hostile. But there may need to be some restriction and channeling of the expression of feelings consistent with our professional responsibilities as clinicians. Our behavior may best be programmed according to the value systems and mutual understanding of the clinician and stutterer. Perhaps we should say that our reactions at such times should be reasonably consistent with previous behaviors displayed in therapy, should relate to the needs of the stutterer and his ability to profit from our expressions of feelings.

the problem of relapses.

In stuttering therapy, as in most other forms of learning, the so-called relapse poses a problem that must be faced and resolved by the clinician. It is easy for us to dismiss a sudden increase of stuttering as inevitable or, on the other hand, to magnify its importance and feel that our therapeutic integrity is threatened. A better response is to attempt to utilize relapses as a validation of the therapy, such as was demonstrated in the case of Alex. The degree to which we can learn to use relapses as part of the therapeutic process is the measure of our freedom from unreasonable fear of them or from the equally inappropriate reaction of treating them as inconsequential. We recognize that progress in stuttering therapy is not steady and that the stutterer frequently regresses in one area when a new step is taken in another. We should not be frightened by this but should learn to use it.

if we only had had more time.

One form of clinical guilt needs special mention. Many clinicians make the assumption that a longer period of therapy would have turned failures into successes. As we examined our case studies, this assumption appears to be erroneous. In some instances, it is possible that excessively long involvement in therapy reinforces failures rather than success and that a shorter, more intensive period may be effective. We are not saying that therapy should not be long-term. The point being made is that as an explanation for failure, the excuse of not having enough time has been overrated.

A closely related and probably equally erroneous assumption is that any interruption in the therapy program before successful termination is harmful. All of us work under schedules that lead to some discontinuity of therapy. Therapy may be interrupted by academic scheduling, by vacations (on either the client's or the therapist's part), and by professional leaves for conventions, to name but a few. Such breaks are inevitable. The wise clinician learns to take advantage of such gaps in the therapy program by proper planning. Lack of continuity in therapy may even be desirable at times, as a way of allowing a stutterer a temporary diversion from concentrated effort or to provide opportunities for self-therapy.

fears of the clinician.

Another barrier to success lies in the myriad fears which the clinician may experience. These occur with all clinicians. All of us are afraid at times of the heavy responsibility that is involved for some cases. When we do not know what to do, the chasm of the unknown yawns before us and we are distressed by confusion and possible failure. If we aren't careful this fear can be transferred to the people we are treating—the stutterer—or his parents. A vicious circle of fear and negative expectation may, therefore, evolve and be transmitted to the stutterer.

the clinician's feelings of guilt.

Anyone who works at helping others is confronted periodically with feelings of guilt—for omissions, imperceptiveness, mistaken judgments, lack of sufficient effort, failure to support a conviction, or inability to understand the stutterer. Such feelings, if they are too intense or chronic, may immobilize the clinician or prevent the optimum growth of which he is capable. Yet, without a modicum of these feelings, we tend to become smug, complacent and static—sure signs that our clinical skills are deteriorating. Thus, it becomes mandatory to find ways to manage the guilt—to handle it constructively as a driving force for improvement and not as a roadblock to development. It helps to admit it openly and to identify its source and character. Such expression may well be followed by looking for ways to avoid the same pitfall in the future. In this way we can convert our guilt feelings into useful learning experiences.

must we always be objective?

The current era of behavioral science sometimes creates confusion. Our frequent assumption is that we must always be objective to be good clinicians. This is impossible when human beings deal with other human beings. We want to be objective, but frequently the lack of factual data or the apparent inconsistency between facts and feelings make us uncomfortable. Sometimes it pays to take a step with an individual simply because it "feels right," even though objective data is missing. It can be helpful to recognize that there are advantages and disadvantages to either an all-subjective or an all-objective approach to therapy. The error of each can be avoided by attempting to increase our awareness of the nature of what we are doing and feeling, while seeking to insure that neither side of the coin remains uppermost too long. Wherever possible, subjective data should be verified by objective facts, as we need to have some kind of a check on our emotional reactions. On the other hand, a willingness to consider thoughtfully the so-called subjective aspects may lead us to an understanding of the objective data.

acceptance of responsibility at the end of therapy.

We talked earlier about the importance of a stutterer's willingness to work at the beginning of therapy. This trait is equally important when formal therapy sessions are terminated. Most successful instances of therapy with stutterers involved persons who substantially accepted responsibility for their own continued improvement. In some of the examples included in this booklet, the successful cases went on to become auxiliary clinicians for other stutterers. The need for this shift from being the receiver of therapy to being an active participant demands that the clinician recognize when and how he should move the stutterer toward independence. Such a shift seems appropriate when the stutterer displays marked reduction in his use of avoidance, tricks, or struggle, when he is reasonably outgoing in his speech, when he voluntarily demonstrates corrective action, and when he expresses a desire to find his own solutions. Such behaviors can indicate that he is beginning to participate actively and constructively in the solution of his own problems—whether they involve speech or other behaviors. This shift to concentration on the stutterer as a clinician is not indicated, however, when there is evidence that the stutterer is using the independent role as a defense against working on his stuttering or when the stutterer's new role interferes with the progress of others.

the importance of the clinician.

With the foregoing emphasis on the traits of the stutterer that affect success and failure, the question might well be raised as to the importance of the role and value of the clinician. Is the successful matching of a stutterer with a clinician accidental? Could anyone else have helped the stutterer just as easily when it was apparent that he was ready to be helped? A review of case studies presented here indicates that the clinician usually played a very positive role. He brings to the therapy situation a special type of knowledge and understanding. He is aware of the appropriateness or inappropriateness of various approaches to the problem. He may well serve as a catalyst, but if this is his only value, many successes would probably not occur. A good relationship with a stutterer is not enough. Most of our cases have already had good relationships with parents, teachers or others important to them at some time in their life. Perhaps it is better to view the clinician as a crucial intervening variable in the therapeutic process. Sometimes he finds it necessary to assume certain roles—sometimes he is assigned certain roles—sometimes he has to achieve certain roles in order to meet the case's needs. Regardless of the specific role, it is only too obvious that his relationship with the stutterer is highly important.

references

1. Bar, A. Analysis of interaction processes during therapy interviews with stutterers, Unpublished Ph.D. dissertation, University of Pittsburgh, 1966.

2. Dollard, J. and Miller, N. *Personality and Psychotherapy.* New York: McGraw-Hill, 1950.

3. Eysenck, H. J. (ed.) *Behavior Therapy and the Neuroses.* London: Pergamon Press, 1960.

4. Fromm-Reichmann, F. *Principles of Intensive Psychotherapy.* Chicago: The University of Chicago Press, 1950.

5. Harrison, S. I. and Clark, D. J. *A Guide to Psychotherapy.* Boston: Little, Brown & Co., 1966.

6. Jourard, S. M. *The Transparent Self.* D. Van Nostrand Company, Inc. 1964.

7. Lennard, H. and Bernstein, A. *The Anatomy of Psychotherapy.* New York: Columbia University Press, 1960.

8. Menninger, K. *Theory of Psychoanalytic Technique.* New York: Basic Books, Inc., 1958.

9. Reik, T. *Listening with the Third Ear.* New York, Harcourt, Brace, 1949.

10. Rogers, C. *On Becoming a Person.* New York: Houghton-Mifflin Co., 1961.

11. Sheehan, J. (chairman), Murphy, A. and Van Riper, C. Successes and Failures in Stuttering Therapy. Symposium, American Speech and Hearing Association Meetings, Chicago, November, 1963.

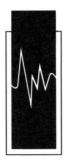The Stuttering Foundation of America is a non-profit charitable organization dedicated to the prevention and improved treatment of stuttering. If you feel that this book has helped you and you wish to help this cause, send a contribution to us at P.O. Box 11749, Memphis, Tennessee 38111-0749. Contributions are tax-deductible.